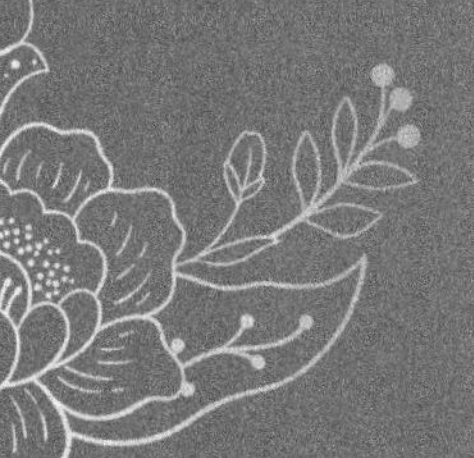

the healthy happy gut menu

Breakfast

Snacks and Appetizers

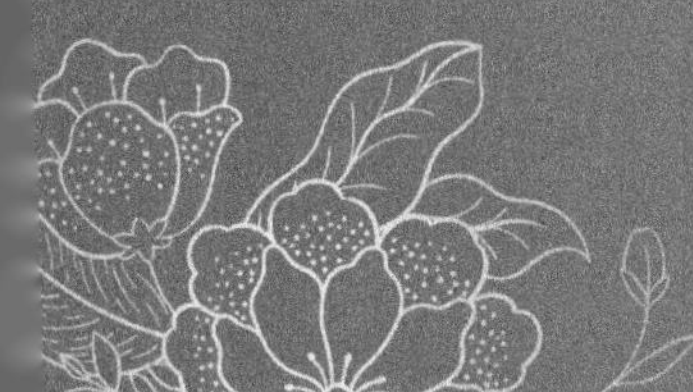
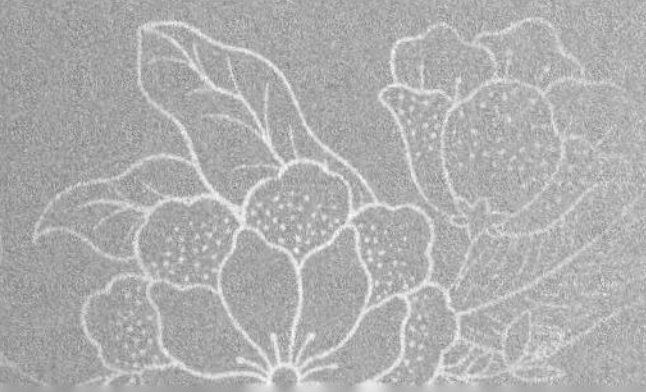

the healthy happy gut menu

Soups and Stews

Main Dishes

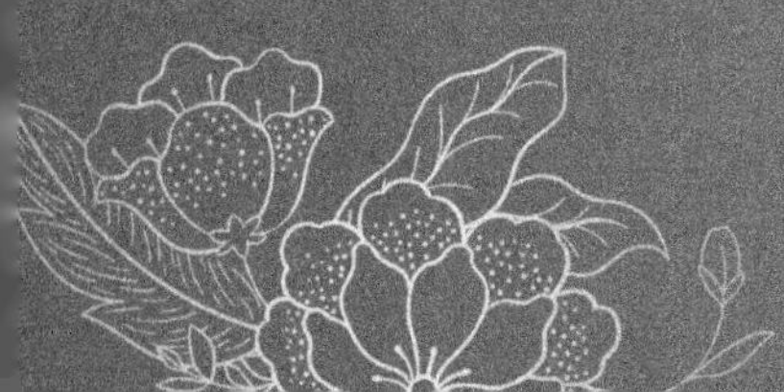
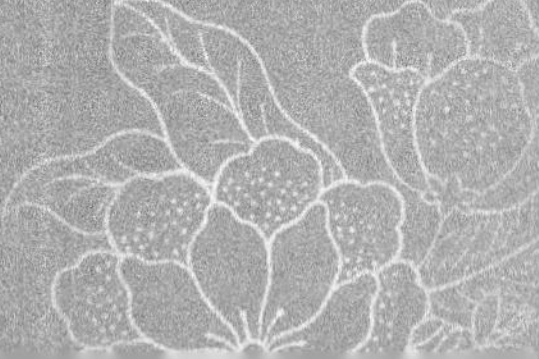

the healthy happy gut menu

Main Dishes

Vegetarian and Vegan Dishes

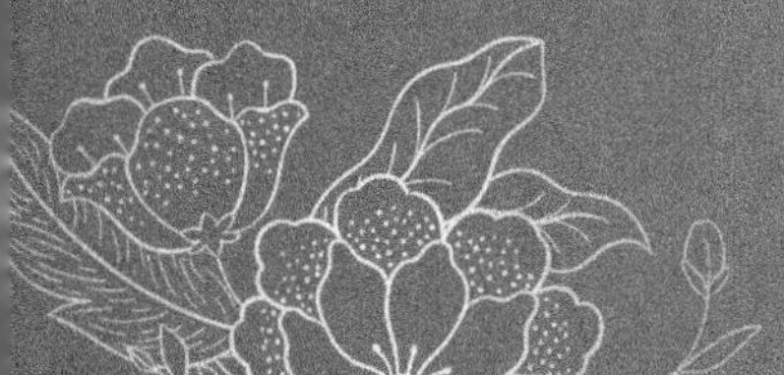
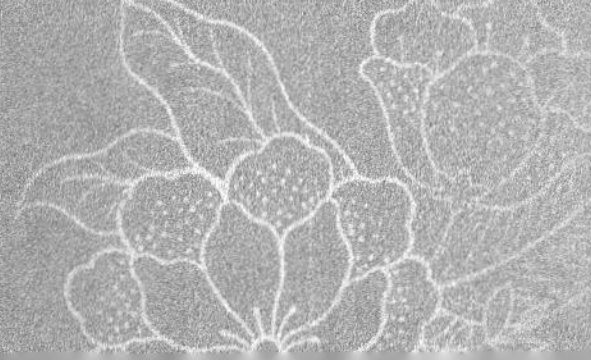

the healthy happy gut menu

Vegetarian and Vegan Dishes

More Dishes (Mixed Categories)

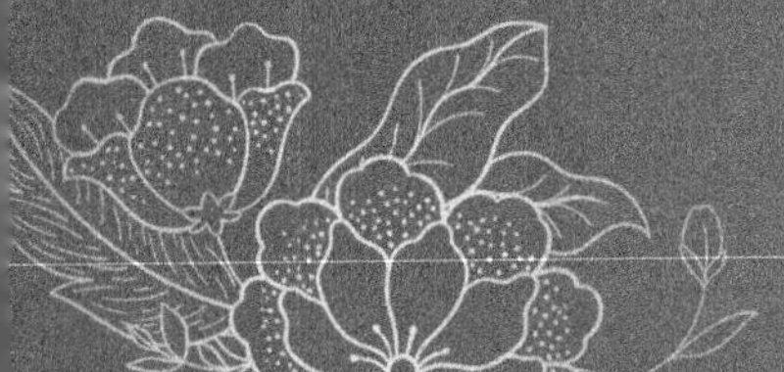

the healthy happy gut menu

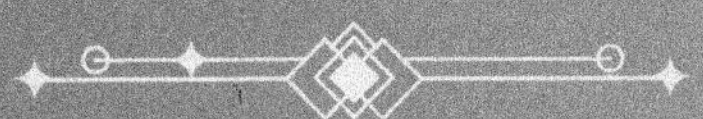

More Dishes (Mixed Categories)

1. Easy Scrambled Eggs

Ingredients:

- 2 large eggs
- 1 tbsp unsalted butter or olive oil
- 1 tbsp milk or cream (optional)
- Salt and pepper to taste

PreparationTime: 5 minutes
Cook Time: 5 minutes
Total Time: 10 minutes
Serves: 1-2 people

Instructions:

1. Crack the eggs into a small bowl and beat them lightly with a fork or whisk until blended. If using, stir in the milk or cream.

2. Heat a small non-stick skillet over medium heat and melt the butter or heat the oil.

3. Pour the egg mixture into the hot pan. As the eggs start to set around the edges, use a spatula to gently push the cooked eggs towards the center, tilting the pan to allow the uncooked egg to flow to the edges.

4. Continue this gentle folding and stirring motion until the eggs are softly scrambled and cooked through, about 2-3 minutes total.

5. Season with salt and pepper to taste.

6. Serve the scrambled eggs immediately while hot.

Tips:
- For creamier scrambled eggs, use a bit more milk or cream.

- Don't overcook the eggs - they should still be moist and tender when served.

- You can also add chopped herbs, cheese, or other fillings to the scrambled eggs.

Enjoy your easy homemade scrambled eggs!

2. Greek Yogurt with Berries

Ingredients:

- 1 cup plain Greek yogurt
- 1/2 cup fresh or frozen berries
 (such as blueberries, raspberries, or strawberries)
- 1 tsp honey (optional)
- 1 tbsp chopped nuts or granola (optional)

PreparationTime: 5 minutes
Cook Time: 0 minutes
Total Time: 5 minutes
Serves: 1 serving

Instructions:

1. Scoop the Greek yogurt into a bowl or serving dish.

2. Top the yogurt with the fresh or frozen berries.

3. If desired, drizzle the honey over the top of the berries.

4. Sprinkle the chopped nuts or granola over the top (if using).

That's it! This simple and healthy snack or breakfast is ready to enjoy.

Tips:
- Use your favorite type of berries or a mix of different berries.

- Adjust the amount of honey to your taste preference.

- Add a sprinkle of cinnamon or a squeeze of lemon juice for extra flavor.

- For a creamier texture, use full-fat Greek yogurt.

- Make it ahead of time and refrigerate until ready to serve.

Enjoy your delicious and nutritious Greek yogurt with berries!

3. Berry Smoothie

Ingredients:

- 1 cup frozen mixed berries
 (such as blueberries, raspberries,
and strawberries)
- 1 cup unsweetened almond milk
 (or milk of your choice)
- 1/2 cup plain Greek yogurt
- 1 tbsp honey (optional)
- 1 tsp vanilla extract (optional)

PreparationTime: 5 minutes
Cook Time: 0 minutes
Total Time: 5 minutes
Serves: 1 serving

Instructions:

1. Add the frozen berries, almond milk, Greek yogurt, honey (if using), and vanilla extract (if using) to a high-speed blender.

2. Blend on high speed until the mixture is smooth and creamy, about 1-2 minutes.

3. Taste and adjust sweetness by adding more honey if desired.

4. Pour the smoothie into a glass and enjoy immediately.

Tips:
- Use a combination of your favorite berries for more flavor.

- Add a handful of spinach or kale for extra nutrients.

- Use plain or vanilla-flavored Greek yogurt.

- Substitute the honey with maple syrup or agave nectar if preferred.

- Add a scoop of protein powder for extra protein.

- Garnish with fresh berries, a sprinkle of cinnamon, or a mint leaf.

Enjoy your refreshing and nutritious berry smoothie!

4. Avocado Toast

Ingredients:

- 1 slice of whole-grain or sourdough bread, toasted
- 1/2 ripe avocado, mashed
- 1 tbsp olive oil
- 1 tsp lemon juice
- Salt and pepper to taste
- Optional toppings: sliced tomatoes, crumbled feta, chopped fresh herbs, red pepper flakes, etc.

PreparationTime: 5 minutes
Cook Time: 0 minutes
Total Time: 5 minutes
Serves: 1 serving

Instructions:

1. Toast the bread until golden brown.

2. In a small bowl, mash the avocado with a fork until it reaches your desired consistency.

3. Add the olive oil and lemon juice to the mashed avocado and mix well.

4. Season the avocado mixture with salt and pepper to taste.

5. Spread the avocado mixture evenly over the toasted bread.

6. Add any desired toppings, such as sliced tomatoes, crumbled feta, chopped fresh herbs, or a sprinkle of red pepper flakes.

7. Serve immediately and enjoy your delicious avocado toast!

Tips:
- Use ripe, creamy avocados for the best flavor and texture.
- Adjust the amount of lemon juice to your taste preference.
- Try different types of bread, such as whole-grain, sourdough, or multigrain.
- Get creative with your toppings - the possibilities are endless!
- For a heartier meal, add a fried or poached egg on top.

Enjoy your healthy and satisfying avocado toast!

5. Cinnamon Oatmeal

Ingredients: Breakfast

- 1/2 cup old-fashioned rolled oats
- 1 cup unsweetened almond milk
 (or milk of your choice)
- 1 tsp ground cinnamon
- 1 tbsp honey (or maple syrup)
- 1/4 tsp vanilla extract
- Pinch of salt

PreparationTime: 5 minutes
Cook Time: 10 minutes
Total Time: 15 minutes
Serves: 1 serving

Optional Toppings:
- Fresh berries
- Chopped nuts or seeds
- Nut butter
- Shredded coconut

Instructions:
1. In a small saucepan, combine the rolled oats and almond milk. Bring the mixture to a simmer over medium heat.

2. Reduce the heat to low and let the oatmeal cook, stirring occasionally, for about 8-10 minutes or until it reaches your desired thickness.

3. Remove the saucepan from the heat and stir in the ground cinnamon, honey (or maple syrup), vanilla extract, and a pinch of salt.

4. Transfer the cinnamon oatmeal to a bowl.

5. Top the oatmeal with your desired toppings, such as fresh berries, chopped nuts or seeds, nut butter, or shredded coconut.

6. Serve the cinnamon oatmeal warm and enjoy!

Tips:
- Use old-fashioned rolled oats for a heartier texture. Quick oats can also be used for a smoother consistency.
- Adjust the amount of milk to achieve your preferred oatmeal consistency.
- Feel free to experiment with different spices, such as nutmeg or cardamom.
- For extra creaminess, stir in a tablespoon of nut butter or Greek yogurt.
- Make it ahead of time and reheat it in the morning for a quick and easy breakfast.

6. Chia Seed Pudding

Ingredients:

- 1/4 cup chia seeds
- 1 cup unsweetened almond milk
(or milk of your choice)
- 1 tbsp honey or maple syrup (optional)
- 1/2 tsp vanilla extract
- Pinch of salt

Optional Toppings:
- Fresh berries
- Chopped nuts or seeds
- Shredded coconut
- Cinnamon

Breakfast

PreparationTime: 10 minutes
Chilling Time: 2-4 hours
Total Time: 2-4 hours 10 minutes
Serves: 2 servings

Instructions:

1. In a medium-sized bowl, whisk together the chia seeds, almond milk, honey or maple syrup (if using), vanilla extract, and a pinch of salt until well combined.

2. Cover the bowl and refrigerate for at least 2-4 hours, or overnight, stirring occasionally, until the chia seeds have thickened the mixture into a pudding-like consistency.

3. Once the chia seed pudding has set, give it a final stir to ensure it's evenly mixed.

4. Divide the chia seed pudding into two serving bowls or jars.

5. Top the pudding with your desired toppings, such as fresh berries, chopped nuts or seeds, shredded coconut, or a sprinkle of cinnamon.

6. Serve chilled and enjoy your delicious chia seed pudding!

Tips:
- Use different types of milk, such as coconut milk or oat milk, for variation.
- Adjust the amount of honey or maple syrup to your desired sweetness level.
- Experiment with different mix-ins, like cocoa powder, peanut butter, or mashed banana.
- Prepare the pudding in advance for a quick and easy breakfast or snack.
- Store any leftover chia seed pudding in the refrigerator for up to 5 days.

7. Spinach and Feta Omelette

Ingredients:

- 3 eggs
- 1 tbsp olive oil or butter
- 1/2 cup fresh spinach, chopped
- 2 tbsp crumbled feta cheese
- Salt and pepper to taste

PreparationTime: 5 minutes
Cook Time: 10 minutes
Total Time: 15 minutes
Serves: 1 serving

Instructions:

1. Crack the eggs into a small bowl and beat them lightly with a fork until well combined.

2. Heat a small non-stick skillet over medium heat and add the olive oil or butter.

3. Once the pan is hot, pour the beaten eggs into the skillet. Let the eggs cook for about 30 seconds to 1 minute, until the edges start to set.

4. Using a spatula, gently push the cooked egg towards the center of the pan, tilting the pan to allow the uncooked egg to flow to the edges. Repeat this process until the eggs are mostly set but still slightly runny in the center, about 2-3 minutes.

5. Sprinkle the chopped spinach and crumbled feta cheese over the top of the eggs.

6. Fold the omelette in half and let it cook for an additional 1-2 minutes, or until the eggs are fully cooked and the cheese is melted.

7. Carefully slide the omelette onto a plate and season with salt and pepper to taste.

8. Serve the spinach and feta omelette hot and enjoy!

Tips:
- Use fresh, high-quality ingredients for the best flavor.
- Adjust the amount of spinach and feta to your personal preference.
- Try adding other fillings, such as diced tomatoes, mushrooms, or onions.
- For a fluffier omelette, separate the egg whites and beat them until stiff before folding them into the yolks.
- Serve the omelette with a side of toast or a fresh salad for a complete meal.

Enjoy your delicious spinach and feta omelette!

8. Almond Butter Banana Toast

Ingredients:

Breakfast

- 1 slice of whole-grain or sourdough bread, toasted
- 2 tbsp creamy almond butter
- 1 ripe banana, sliced
- Drizzle of honey (optional)
- Sprinkle of cinnamon (optional)

PreparationTime: 5 minutes
Cook Time: 0 minutes
Total Time: 5 minutes
Serves: 1 serving

Instructions:

1. Toast the slice of bread until it's golden brown.

2. Spread the almond butter evenly over the toasted bread.

3. Arrange the sliced banana on top of the almond butter.

4. If desired, drizzle a small amount of honey over the banana slices.

5. Sprinkle a light dusting of cinnamon over the top (optional).

That's it! Your delicious and nutritious almond butter banana toast is ready to enjoy.

Tips:
- Use ripe, sweet bananas for the best flavor.

- Substitute the almond butter with peanut butter or another nut butter if preferred.

- Add a sprinkle of chopped nuts or seeds for extra crunch.

- For a heartier meal, serve the toast with a side of fresh fruit or a hard-boiled egg.

- Make it ahead of time and pack it for a quick and easy breakfast or snack on the go.

Enjoy your tasty and satisfying almond butter banana toast!

9. Cottage Cheese with Pineapple

Ingredients:

- 1/2 cup low-fat or full-fat cottage cheese
- 1/2 cup fresh pineapple chunks
- 1 tsp honey (optional)
- Sprinkle of cinnamon (optional)

PreparationTime: 5 minutes
Cook Time: 0 minutes
Total Time: 5 minutes
Serves: 1 serving

Instructions:

1. Scoop the cottage cheese into a small bowl or serving dish.

2. Top the cottage cheese with the fresh pineapple chunks.

3. If desired, drizzle the honey over the pineapple and cottage cheese.

4. Sprinkle a light dusting of cinnamon over the top (optional).

That's it! Your simple and refreshing cottage cheese with pineapple is ready to enjoy.

Tips:
- Use canned pineapple chunks if fresh pineapple is not available.

- Adjust the amount of honey to your taste preference.

- Try adding other fresh fruit, such as berries or diced mango, for variety.

- For a creamier texture, use full-fat cottage cheese.

- Serve the cottage cheese and pineapple as a snack or light breakfast.

- Make it ahead of time and refrigerate until ready to serve.

Enjoy your delicious and nutritious cottage cheese with pineapple!

10. Ham and Cheese Roll-Ups

Ingredients:

Breakfast

- 8 slices of deli ham
- 4 slices of cheddar or Swiss cheese
- 2 tbsp cream cheese, softened
- 1 tbsp Dijon mustard
- 1 tsp dried parsley (optional)
- Salt and pepper to taste

PreparationTime: 10 minutes
Cook Time: 0 minutes
Total Time: 10 minutes
Serves: 4 servings (2 roll-ups each)

Instructions:

1. Lay the slices of deli ham flat on a clean work surface.

2. In a small bowl, mix together the softened cream cheese and Dijon mustard until well combined.

3. Spread a thin layer of the cream cheese mixture evenly over each slice of ham.

4. Place a slice of cheese on top of the cream cheese mixture on each ham slice.

5. Carefully roll up each ham slice tightly, starting from one of the short ends and rolling towards the other end.

6. Sprinkle the dried parsley (if using) over the top of the rolled-up ham and cheese.

7. Season with a pinch of salt and pepper.

8. Cut each rolled-up ham and cheese in half to create 8 roll-ups.

9. Serve the ham and cheese roll-ups immediately or refrigerate until ready to serve.

Tips:
- Use your favorite types of deli ham and cheese.
- Adjust the amount of cream cheese and mustard to your taste preference.
- Try adding a thin slice of tomato or a few spinach leaves for extra flavor and nutrition.
- For a crunchier texture, sprinkle the roll-ups with crushed crackers or breadcrumbs before serving.
- These roll-ups make a great snack, appetizer, or light lunch.

Enjoy your delicious and easy-to-make ham and cheese roll-ups!

11. Veggie Sticks with Hummus

Ingredients:

- 1 cup assorted fresh vegetables,
cut into sticks (such as carrots, celery,
 cucumber, bell peppers)
- 1/2 cup hummus (store-bought or homemade)

PreparationTime: 10 minutes
Cook Time: 0 minutes
Total Time: 10 minutes
Serves: 2-3 servings

Optional Toppings:
- Chopped fresh herbs (parsley, cilantro, or dill)
- Sprinkle of paprika or za'atar seasoning
- Drizzle of olive oil

Instructions:

1. Wash and prepare the assorted fresh vegetables. Cut them into long, thin sticks or slices, about 4-6 inches long.

2. Arrange the veggie sticks on a serving plate or platter.

3. Scoop the hummus into a small bowl or ramekin and place it in the center of the plate, surrounded by the veggie sticks.

4. If desired, sprinkle the hummus with chopped fresh herbs, a light dusting of paprika or za'atar seasoning, and/or a drizzle of olive oil.

5. Serve the veggie sticks with the hummus immediately, or cover and refrigerate until ready to serve.

Tips:
- Choose a variety of colorful vegetables for a visually appealing presentation.
- Adjust the amount of hummus based on the number of servings and your personal preference.
- Try different flavors of hummus, such as roasted red pepper or garlic, for variety.
- Serve the veggie sticks and hummus as a healthy snack, appetizer, or side dish.
- For a heartier meal, pair the veggie sticks and hummus with whole-grain crackers or pita bread.
- Store any leftover hummus in an airtight container in the refrigerator for up to 5 days.

Enjoy your refreshing and nutritious veggie sticks with creamy hummus!

12. Cheese and Apple Slices

Ingredients:

- 1 medium-sized apple, cored and sliced
- 2-3 slices of your favorite cheese
 (such as cheddar, gouda, or brie)
- Optional: Drizzle of honey or sprinkle of cinnamon

PreparationTime: 5 minutes
Cook Time: 0 minutes
Total Time: 5 minutes
Serves: 1 serving

Instructions:

1. Wash and core the apple, then slice it into thin, even slices.

2. Arrange the apple slices on a plate or serving board.

3. Place the cheese slices on top of the apple slices.

4. If desired, drizzle a small amount of honey over the cheese and apple slices.

5. Optionally, sprinkle a light dusting of cinnamon over the top.

That's it! Your simple and delicious cheese and apple slices are ready to enjoy.

Tips:
- Choose a crisp, tart apple variety, such as Granny Smith or Honeycrisp, for the best flavor contrast with the cheese.

- Experiment with different types of cheese, such as brie, gouda, or sharp cheddar, to find your favorite pairing.

- For a more substantial snack, serve the cheese and apple slices with a few whole-grain crackers or a small handful of nuts.

- Prepare the apple slices just before serving to prevent them from browning.

- Store any leftover apple slices in an airtight container in the refrigerator for up to 3 days.

Enjoy your simple and satisfying cheese and apple slices!

13. Almond Clusters

Ingredients:

- 1 cup raw almonds
- 1/4 cup honey
- 1 tbsp coconut oil
- 1/4 tsp sea salt

PreparationTime: 10 minutes
Cook Time: 15 minutes
Total Time: 25 minutes
Serves: 12 clusters

Instructions:

1. Preheat your oven to 325°F (165°C) and line a baking sheet with parchment paper.

2. In a medium-sized bowl, combine the raw almonds, honey, coconut oil, and sea salt. Stir until the almonds are evenly coated.

3. Scoop the almond mixture by the tablespoonful and place them onto the prepared baking sheet, spacing them a few inches apart.

4. Bake the almond clusters in the preheated oven for 12-15 minutes, or until they are golden brown and fragrant.

5. Remove the baking sheet from the oven and let the almond clusters cool completely on the sheet, about 10 minutes.

6. Once cooled, gently transfer the almond clusters to an airtight container or storage bag.

Tips:
- Use raw, unsalted almonds for the best flavor and texture.
- Adjust the amount of honey and salt to your taste preference.
- For a chunkier texture, roughly chop the almonds before mixing with the other ingredients.
- Try adding a pinch of cinnamon or a splash of vanilla extract for extra flavor.
- Store the almond clusters in an airtight container at room temperature for up to 1 week.
- These clusters make a great snack, topping for yogurt or oatmeal, or addition to trail mixes.

Enjoy your homemade, crunchy almond clusters!

14. Cucumber Bites

Ingredients:

- 1 medium cucumber, sliced into 12 rounds
- 2 oz cream cheese, softened
- 2 tbsp crumbled feta cheese
- 1 tbsp chopped fresh dill (or 1 tsp dried dill)
- Salt and pepper to taste

PreparationTime: 10 minutes
Cook Time: 0 minutes
Total Time: 10 minutes
Serves: 12 bites

Instructions:

1. Slice the cucumber into 12 even rounds, about 1/4 inch thick.

2. In a small bowl, mix together the softened cream cheese, crumbled feta cheese, and chopped fresh dill (or dried dill) until well combined.

3. Spread or pipe a small amount of the cream cheese mixture onto each cucumber round.

4. Season the cucumber bites with a pinch of salt and pepper.

5. Arrange the cucumber bites on a serving platter or plate.

6. Refrigerate the cucumber bites until ready to serve.

Tips:
- Use an English or Persian cucumber for the best texture and flavor.
- For a creamier filling

15. Deviled Eggs

Ingredients:

- 6 hard-boiled eggs
- 2 tbsp mayonnaise
- 1 tsp Dijon mustard
- 1 tsp white vinegar
- 1/4 tsp paprika
- Salt and pepper to taste
- Chopped chives or parsley for garnish (optional)

PreparationTime: 15 minutes
Cook Time: 15 minutes
Total Time: 30 minutes
Serves: 12 deviled eggs

Instructions:

1. Place the hard-boiled eggs in a bowl of cold water and let them sit for 5 minutes. This will make them easier to peel.

2. Peel the eggs and cut them in half lengthwise.

3. Carefully remove the yolks from the egg whites and place the yolks in a small bowl.

4. Add the mayonnaise, Dijon mustard, white vinegar, and a pinch of salt and pepper to the bowl with the egg yolks. Mash and mix everything together until smooth and creamy.

5. Using a spoon or a piping bag, fill the egg white halves with the yolk mixture.

6. Sprinkle the deviled eggs with paprika for a touch of color.

7. Optionally, garnish the deviled eggs with chopped chives or parsley.

8. Refrigerate the deviled eggs until ready to serve.

Tips:
- For the creamiest filling, use room temperature eggs and mayonnaise.
- Experiment with different seasonings, such as cayenne pepper, garlic powder, or chopped pickles.
- Refrigerate the deviled eggs for at least 30 minutes before serving to allow the flavors to meld.
- Store any leftover deviled eggs in an airtight container in the refrigerator for up to 3 days.

Enjoy your delicious and classic deviled eggs!

16. Turkey and Cheese Roll-Ups

Ingredients:

- 8 slices of deli turkey
- 4 slices of cheddar or Swiss cheese
- 2 tbsp cream cheese, softened
- 1 tbsp Dijon mustard
- 1 tsp dried parsley (optional)
- Salt and pepper to taste

PreparationTime: 10 minutes
Cook Time: 0 minutes
Total Time: 10 minutes
Serves: 4 servings (2 roll-ups each)

Instructions:

1. Lay the slices of deli turkey flat on a clean work surface.

2. In a small bowl, mix together the softened cream cheese and Dijon mustard until well combined.

3. Spread a thin layer of the cream cheese mixture evenly over each slice of turkey.

4. Place a slice of cheese on top of the cream cheese mixture on each turkey slice.

5. Carefully roll up each turkey slice tightly, starting from one of the short ends and rolling towards the other end.

6. Sprinkle the dried parsley (if using) over the top of the rolled-up turkey and cheese.

7. Season with a pinch of salt and pepper.

8. Cut each rolled-up turkey and cheese in half to create 8 roll-ups.

9. Serve the turkey and cheese roll-ups immediately or refrigerate until ready to serve.

Tips:
- Use your favorite types of deli turkey and cheese.
- Adjust the amount of cream cheese and mustard to your taste preference.
- Try adding a thin slice of tomato or a few spinach leaves for extra flavor and nutrition.
- For a crunchier texture, sprinkle the roll-ups with crushed crackers or breadcrumbs before serving.
- These roll-ups make a great snack, appetizer, or light lunch.

Enjoy your delicious and easy-to-make turkey and cheese roll-ups!

17. Caprese Skewers

Ingredients:

- 12 cherry or grape tomatoes
- 12 small fresh mozzarella balls (or cubes)
- 12 fresh basil leaves
- 2 tbsp balsamic glaze
- 1 tbsp extra-virgin olive oil
- Salt and pepper to taste

PreparationTime: 15 minutes
Cook Time: 0 minutes
Total Time: 15 minutes
Serves: 12 skewers

Instructions:

1. Thread the ingredients onto 12 small skewers or toothpicks, alternating between a tomato, a mozzarella ball, and a basil leaf.

2. Arrange the Caprese skewers on a serving platter or board.

3. Drizzle the balsamic glaze and olive oil over the skewers.

4. Season with a pinch of salt and pepper.

5. Serve the Caprese skewers immediately or refrigerate until ready to serve.

Tips:
- Use the freshest, ripest tomatoes and highest-quality mozzarella for the best flavor.

- For a more substantial appetizer, use larger cherry tomatoes and mozzarella balls.

- Substitute the balsamic glaze with a balsamic vinegar reduction or regular balsamic vinegar.

- Add a sprinkle of dried Italian seasoning or a pinch of red pepper flakes for extra flavor.

- Refrigerate any leftover Caprese skewers in an airtight container for up to 2 days.

- Serve the Caprese skewers as an appetizer, side dish, or light snack.

Enjoy your fresh and flavorful Caprese skewers!

18. Greek Yogurt with Honey

Ingredients:

- 1 cup plain Greek yogurt
- 1-2 tbsp honey
- Optional toppings: granola,
  fresh fruit, nuts, cinnamon

Snacks and Appetizers

PreparationTime: 5 minutes
Cook Time: 0 minutes
Total Time: 5 minutes
Serves: 1 serving

Instructions:

1. Scoop the plain Greek yogurt into a bowl or serving dish.

2. Drizzle the honey over the top of the yogurt, using 1-2 tablespoons depending on your desired sweetness level.

3. If desired, add any optional toppings such as granola, fresh fruit (e.g., berries, sliced bananas, diced mango), chopped nuts, or a sprinkle of cinnamon.

4. Gently stir the honey into the yogurt until it's well combined.

5. Serve the Greek yogurt with honey immediately, or refrigerate until ready to enjoy.

Tips:
- Use full-fat or low-fat Greek yogurt, depending on your preference.

- Adjust the amount of honey to your taste - start with 1 tablespoon and add more if you want it sweeter.

- Try different types of honey, such as wildflower, clover, or raw honey, for variety.

- For a creamier texture, use a thicker, higher-protein Greek yogurt.

- Add a sprinkle of chia seeds, flaxseeds, or shredded coconut for extra nutrition and crunch.

- This makes a great breakfast, snack, or healthy dessert.

Enjoy your simple and delicious Greek yogurt with honey!

19. Roasted Chickpeas

Ingredients:

- 1 (15 oz) can chickpeas, drained and rinsed
- 1 tbsp olive oil
- 1 tsp ground cumin
- 1 tsp paprika
- 1/2 tsp garlic powder
- 1/4 tsp salt
- 1/4 tsp black pepper

Snacks and Appetizers

PreparationTime: 10 minutes
Cook Time: 25-30 minutes
Total Time: 35-40 minutes
Serves: 4 servings

Instructions:

1. Preheat your oven to 400°F (200°C).

2. Drain and rinse the chickpeas, then pat them dry with a paper towel or clean kitchen towel.

3. In a medium-sized bowl, toss the chickpeas with the olive oil, cumin, paprika, garlic powder, salt, and black pepper until the chickpeas are evenly coated.

4. Spread the seasoned chickpeas in a single layer on a baking sheet lined with parchment paper.

5. Roast the chickpeas in the preheated oven for 25-30 minutes, stirring halfway, until they are crispy and golden brown.

6. Remove the roasted chickpeas from the oven and let them cool for a few minutes before serving.

Tips:
- For extra crispiness, pat the chickpeas very dry before seasoning.
- Adjust the spices to your taste preferences - try adding cayenne pepper for a spicy kick.
- Experiment with different seasoning blends, such as chili powder, lemon pepper, or Italian herbs.
- Roast the chickpeas in batches if needed to ensure they have enough space to crisp up.
- Store any leftover roasted chickpeas in an airtight container at room temperature for up to 5 days.
- Enjoy the roasted chickpeas as a snack, salad topping, or addition to grain bowls.

20. Celery Sticks with Peanut Butter

Ingredients:

Snacks and Appetizers

- 2-3 celery stalks, cut into 4-inch sticks
- 2-3 tbsp creamy peanut butter
- Optional toppings: raisins, chopped nuts, honey

PreparationTime: 5 minutes
Cook Time: 0 minutes
Total Time: 5 minutes
Serves: 1 serving

Instructions:

1. Wash the celery stalks and cut them into 4-inch sticks.

2. Spread a generous amount of peanut butter onto each celery stick, using about 2-3 tablespoons total.

3. If desired, top the peanut butter-filled celery sticks with any of the optional toppings, such as raisins, chopped nuts, or a drizzle of honey.

4. Arrange the celery sticks with peanut butter on a plate or in a serving dish.

5. Serve immediately or refrigerate until ready to enjoy.

Tips:
- Use crunchy peanut butter for added texture, or creamy peanut butter for a smoother filling.
- Try other nut or seed butters, such as almond butter or sunflower seed butter, for variety.
- Cut the celery sticks to your desired length, keeping them long enough to hold the peanut butter.
- For a healthier option, use natural or organic peanut butter without added sugars or oils.
- Pair the celery sticks with peanut butter as a snack, appetizer, or part of a balanced meal.
- Store any leftover celery sticks with peanut butter in an airtight container in the refrigerator for up to 3 days.

Enjoy your simple and nutritious celery sticks with peanut butter!

21. Tomato Basil Soup

Ingredients:

- 2 tbsp olive oil
- 1 onion, diced
- 3 cloves garlic, minced
- 1 (28 oz) can crushed tomatoes
- 2 cups vegetable or chicken broth
- 1/4 cup fresh basil leaves, chopped
- 1 tsp dried oregano
- 1 tsp sugar
- Salt and pepper to taste
- Heavy cream or half-and-half (optional)

PreparationTime: 15 minutes
Cook Time: 30 minutes
Total Time: 45 minutes
Serves: 4 servings

Instructions:

1. In a large saucepan or Dutch oven, heat the olive oil over medium heat. Add the diced onion and sauté for 5-7 minutes, until the onion is translucent.

2. Add the minced garlic and sauté for an additional 1-2 minutes, until fragrant.

3. Pour in the can of crushed tomatoes and the vegetable or chicken broth. Stir to combine.

4. Add the chopped fresh basil, dried oregano, and sugar. Season with salt and pepper to taste.

5. Bring the soup to a simmer and let it cook for 20-25 minutes, stirring occasionally, until the flavors have melded and the soup has thickened slightly.

6. If desired, stir in a splash of heavy cream or half-and-half to make the soup creamier.

7. Serve the tomato basil soup hot, garnished with additional fresh basil leaves if desired.

Tips:
- Use high-quality canned crushed tomatoes for the best flavor.
- Adjust the amount of broth to achieve your desired consistency.
- For a smoother soup, use an immersion blender or regular blender to puree the soup before adding the cream.
- Pair the tomato basil soup with grilled cheese sandwiches, crusty bread, or a fresh salad for a complete meal.
- Refrigerate any leftover soup in an airtight container for up to 4 days.

22. Chicken Vegetable Soup

Ingredients:

- 1 lb boneless, skinless chicken breasts, cubed
- 2 tbsp olive oil
- 1 onion, diced
- 3 carrots, peeled and sliced
- 3 celery stalks, sliced
- 3 cloves garlic, minced
- 6 cups low-sodium chicken broth
- 1 (15 oz) can diced tomatoes
- 1 cup frozen peas
- 1 cup frozen corn
- 1 tsp dried thyme
- 1 tsp dried parsley
- Salt and pepper to taste

PreparationTime: 20 minutes
Cook Time: 45 minutes
Total Time: 1 hour 5 minutes
Serves: 6 servings

Instructions:

1. In a large pot or Dutch oven, heat the olive oil over medium-high heat. Add the cubed chicken and cook until lightly browned, about 5-7 minutes. Remove the chicken from the pot and set aside.

2. In the same pot, add the diced onion, sliced carrots, and sliced celery. Sauté for 5-7 minutes, until the vegetables start to soften.

3. Add the minced garlic and sauté for an additional 1-2 minutes, until fragrant.

4. Pour in the chicken broth and diced tomatoes. Bring the mixture to a boil.

5. Once boiling, reduce the heat to medium-low and let the soup simmer for 20 minutes.

6. Add the cooked chicken, frozen peas, frozen corn, dried thyme, and dried parsley. Season with salt and pepper to taste.

7. Continue simmering the soup for an additional 15-20 minutes, or until the vegetables are tender and the flavors have melded.

8. Serve the chicken vegetable soup hot, garnished with additional fresh parsley if desired.

23. Lentil Stew

Ingredients:

- 1 tbsp olive oil
- 1 onion, diced
- 3 cloves garlic, minced
- 2 carrots, peeled and diced
- 2 celery stalks, diced
- 1 cup dried brown or green lentils, rinsed
- 4 cups low-sodium vegetable or chicken broth
- 1 (14.5 oz) can diced tomatoes
- 2 tsp dried thyme
- 1 tsp dried rosemary
- 1 bay leaf
- Salt and pepper to taste
- Chopped parsley for garnish (optional)

PreparationTime: 15 minutes
Cook Time: 45 minutes
Total Time: 1 hour
Serves: 4-6 servings

Instructions:

1. In a large pot or Dutch oven, heat the olive oil over medium heat. Add the diced onion and sauté for 5-7 minutes, until translucent.

2. Add the minced garlic and sauté for an additional 1-2 minutes, until fragrant.

3. Stir in the diced carrots and celery. Sauté for 3-5 minutes, until the vegetables start to soften.

4. Add the rinsed lentils, vegetable or chicken broth, diced tomatoes, dried thyme, dried rosemary, and bay leaf. Stir to combine.

5. Bring the stew to a boil, then reduce the heat to medium-low and let it simmer for 35-45 minutes, or until the lentils are tender and the stew has thickened.

6. Remove the bay leaf. Season the lentil stew with salt and pepper to taste. Serve the lentil stew hot, garnished with chopped parsley if desired. Enjoy with crusty bread or a side salad.

Tips:
- Use brown or green lentils for a heartier texture. Red lentils will break down more and create a creamier stew.
- Adjust the amount of broth to achieve your desired consistency.

24. Broccoli Cheese Soup

Ingredients:

- 4 cups fresh broccoli florets
- 2 cups low-sodium chicken or vegetable broth
- 1 cup shredded low-fat cheddar cheese
- 1/2 cup unsweetened almond milk

PreparationTime: 10 minutes
Cook Time: 20 minutes
Total Time: 30 minutes
Serves: 4 servings

Instructions:

1. In a large saucepan, bring the broth to a boil over medium-high heat.

2. Add the broccoli florets to the boiling broth, reduce the heat to medium-low, and simmer for 10-15 minutes, or until the broccoli is tender.

3. Using an immersion blender or a regular blender, puree the broccoli and broth until smooth.

4. Return the pureed soup to the saucepan and stir in the shredded low-fat cheddar cheese and unsweetened almond milk.

5. Cook the soup over medium heat, stirring frequently, until the cheese is melted and the soup is heated through, about 5 minutes.

6. Serve the broccoli cheese soup hot.

Tips:
- Use fresh broccoli for the best flavor and texture. Frozen broccoli can also be used, but may require a slightly longer cooking time.
- Opt for low-fat or reduced-fat cheddar cheese to keep the soup diabetes-friendly.
- Unsweetened almond milk adds creaminess without the extra carbs and calories of regular milk or cream.
- For a thicker soup, you can blend a portion of the cooked broccoli and then stir it back into the remaining soup.
- Season with a pinch of salt and pepper to taste, if desired.
- Garnish with a sprinkle of extra shredded cheese or a few broccoli florets.

This broccoli cheese soup is a delicious and diabetes-friendly option that's easy to make with just 4 simple ingredients. Enjoy!

25. Beef and Barley Stew

Ingredients:

- 1 lb lean beef stew meat, cubed
- 1 cup pearl barley, rinsed
- 4 cups low-sodium beef broth
- 1 (14.5 oz) can diced tomatoes

PreparationTime: 15 minutes
Cook Time: 1 hour 30 minutes
Total Time: 1 hour 45 minutes
Serves: 4 servings

Instructions:

1. In a large pot or Dutch oven, brown the cubed beef over medium-high heat until no longer pink, about 5-7 minutes. Drain any excess fat.

2. Add the rinsed pearl barley, low-sodium beef broth, and diced tomatoes (with their juices) to the pot. Stir to combine.

3. Bring the stew to a boil, then reduce the heat to low, cover, and simmer for 1 to 1.5 hours, or until the barley is tender and the beef is very tender.

4. Taste the stew and adjust seasoning as needed. You can add a pinch of salt and pepper, if desired.

5. Serve the beef and barley stew hot.

Tips:
- Use lean beef stew meat to keep the fat and calorie content low for a diabetic-friendly meal.
- Pearl barley is a great source of fiber and adds heartiness to the stew.
- Low-sodium beef broth helps control the sodium intake.
- The diced tomatoes provide flavor and additional nutrients.
- For a thicker stew, you can remove the lid during the last 30 minutes of simmering to allow some of the liquid to evaporate.
- Garnish with chopped fresh parsley or chives, if desired.
- Serve the stew with a side salad or steamed vegetables for a complete diabetic-friendly meal.

This simple 4-ingredient beef and barley stew is a comforting and diabetes-friendly option that's easy to prepare. Enjoy!

26. Carrot Ginger Soup

Ingredients:

Soups and Stews

- 1 tbsp olive oil
- 1 onion, diced
- 3 cloves garlic, minced
- 1 lb carrots, peeled and sliced
- 1 tbsp grated fresh ginger
- 4 cups low-sodium vegetable or chicken broth
- 1 tsp ground cumin
- 1/4 tsp cayenne pepper (optional)
- Salt and pepper to taste
- Chopped fresh cilantro for garnish (optional)

PreparationTime: 15 minutes
Cook Time: 30 minutes
Total Time: 45 minutes
Serves: 4 servings

Instructions:

1. In a large pot or Dutch oven, heat the olive oil over medium heat. Add the diced onion and sauté for 5-7 minutes, until translucent.

2. Add the minced garlic and grated ginger. Sauté for an additional 1-2 minutes, until fragrant.

3. Add the sliced carrots, vegetable or chicken broth, ground cumin, and cayenne pepper (if using). Stir to combine.

4. Bring the soup to a boil, then reduce the heat to medium-low and let it simmer for 20-25 minutes, or until the carrots are very tender.

5. Using an immersion blender or a regular blender, puree the soup until smooth.

6. Return the pureed soup to the pot and season with salt and pepper to taste.

7. Serve the carrot ginger soup hot, garnished with chopped fresh cilantro if desired.

Tips:
- Use fresh, high-quality carrots for the best flavor.
- Adjust the amount of ginger to your taste preference.
- For a creamier soup, stir in a splash of heavy cream or coconut milk at the end.
- Add a dollop of plain Greek yogurt or a sprinkle of toasted nuts or seeds for extra texture and flavor.
- Refrigerate any leftover soup in an airtight container for up to 4 days.

27. Mushroom Soup

Ingredients:

- 2 tbsp olive oil
- 1 onion, diced
- 8 oz cremini or button mushrooms, sliced
- 3 cloves garlic, minced
- 2 tbsp all-purpose flour
- 4 cups low-sodium vegetable or chicken broth
- 1 cup unsweetened almond milk
- 1 tsp dried thyme
- Salt and pepper to taste
- Chopped fresh parsley for garnish (optional)

PreparationTime: 15 minutes
Cook Time: 30 minutes
Total Time: 45 minutes
Serves: 4 servings

Instructions:

1. In a large pot or Dutch oven, heat the olive oil over medium heat. Add the diced onion and sauté for 5-7 minutes, until translucent.

2. Add the sliced mushrooms and minced garlic. Sauté for an additional 5-7 minutes, until the mushrooms are softened and the garlic is fragrant.

3. Sprinkle the all-purpose flour over the mushroom mixture and stir to coat the vegetables. Cook for 2-3 minutes, stirring constantly, to cook off the raw flour taste.

4. Gradually pour in the low-sodium vegetable or chicken broth, whisking constantly to prevent lumps from forming.

5. Stir in the unsweetened almond milk and dried thyme. Bring the soup to a simmer and let it cook for 15-20 minutes, stirring occasionally, until the soup has thickened.

6. Season the mushroom soup with salt and pepper to taste.

7. Serve the soup hot, garnished with chopped fresh parsley if desired.

Tips:
- Use a variety of mushrooms, such as cremini, button, and shiitake, for more complex flavor.
- For a creamier soup, use half-and-half or heavy cream instead of almond milk.
- Add a splash of dry sherry or white wine for extra depth of flavor.
- Blend a portion of the soup with an immersion blender for a thicker, creamier texture.
- Refrigerate any leftover soup in an airtight container for up to 4 days.

28. Pumpkin Soup

Ingredients:

- 1 tbsp olive oil
- 1 onion, diced
- 3 cloves garlic, minced
- 1 (15 oz) can pumpkin puree
- 4 cups low-sodium vegetable or chicken broth
- 1 tsp ground cinnamon
- 1/2 tsp ground ginger
- 1/4 tsp ground nutmeg
- Salt and pepper to taste
- Chopped fresh parsley or chives for garnish (optional)

PreparationTime: 15 minutes
Cook Time: 30 minutes
Total Time: 45 minutes
Serves: 4 servings

Instructions:

1. In a large pot or Dutch oven, heat the olive oil over medium heat. Add the diced onion and sauté for 5-7 minutes, until translucent.

2. Add the minced garlic and sauté for an additional 1-2 minutes, until fragrant.

3. Stir in the pumpkin puree, low-sodium vegetable or chicken broth, ground cinnamon, ground ginger, and ground nutmeg. Whisk to combine.

4. Bring the soup to a simmer and let it cook for 20-25 minutes, stirring occasionally, until the flavors have melded.

5. Using an immersion blender or a regular blender, puree the soup until smooth.

6. Return the pureed soup to the pot and season with salt and pepper to taste.

7. Serve the pumpkin soup hot, garnished with chopped fresh parsley or chives if desired.

Tips:
- Use pure pumpkin puree, not pumpkin pie filling, for the best flavor.
- Adjust the spices to your taste preference. You can add more or less cinnamon, ginger, and nutmeg.
- For a creamier soup, stir in a splash of heavy cream or coconut milk at the end.
- Top the soup with roasted pumpkin seeds, croutons, or a dollop of plain Greek yogurt for extra texture and flavor.
- Refrigerate any leftover soup in an airtight container for up to 4 days.

29. Cauliflower Soup

Ingredients:

- 1 tbsp olive oil
- 1 onion, diced
- 3 cloves garlic, minced
- 1 head of cauliflower, cut into florets
- 4 cups low-sodium vegetable or chicken broth
- 1 cup unsweetened almond milk
- 1 tsp dried thyme
- Salt and pepper to taste
- Chopped fresh parsley for garnish (optional)

PreparationTime: 15 minutes
Cook Time: 30 minutes
Total Time: 45 minutes
Serves: 4 servings

Instructions:

1. In a large pot or Dutch oven, heat the olive oil over medium heat. Add the diced onion and sauté for 5-7 minutes, until translucent.

2. Add the minced garlic and sauté for an additional 1-2 minutes, until fragrant.

3. Add the cauliflower florets and the low-sodium vegetable or chicken broth to the pot. Bring the mixture to a boil.

4. Reduce the heat to medium-low and let the soup simmer for 20-25 minutes, or until the cauliflower is very tender.

5. Using an immersion blender or a regular blender, puree the soup until smooth.

6. Return the pureed soup to the pot and stir in the unsweetened almond milk and dried thyme.

7. Season the cauliflower soup with salt and pepper to taste.

8. Serve the soup hot, garnished with chopped fresh parsley if desired.

Tips:
- Use fresh, high-quality cauliflower for the best flavor.
- For a creamier soup, use half-and-half or heavy cream instead of almond milk.
- Add a pinch of nutmeg or a splash of lemon juice for extra flavor.
- Top the soup with roasted cauliflower florets, croutons, or shredded cheese for added texture and taste.
- Refrigerate any leftover soup in an airtight container for up to 4 days.

30. Split Pea Soup

Ingredients:

- 1 lb split peas, rinsed
- 8 cups chicken or vegetable broth
- 1 onion, diced
- 2 carrots, peeled and diced
- 2 celery stalks, diced
- 3 cloves garlic, minced
- 1 bay leaf
- 1 tsp dried thyme
- Salt and pepper to taste

PreparationTime: 15 minutes
Cook Time: 1 hour 15 minutes
Total Time: 1 hour 30 minutes
Serves: 6-8 servings

Instructions:

1. In a large pot, combine the split peas and broth. Bring to a boil over high heat.

2. Reduce heat to medium-low, cover and simmer for 30 minutes, stirring occasionally.

3. Add the onion, carrots, celery, garlic, bay leaf and thyme. Continue simmering, uncovered, for 45-60 minutes, until the peas are very soft and the soup has thickened.

4. Remove the bay leaf. Use an immersion blender to partially puree the soup, leaving some texture.

5. Season with salt and pepper to taste.

6. Serve hot, garnished with croutons, chopped parsley or a swirl of yogurt if desired.

The long simmering time allows the split peas to break down and thicken the soup naturally. Adjust the consistency to your liking by pureeing more or less. Enjoy this hearty, comforting split pea soup!

31. Lemon Herb Chicken

Ingredients:

- 4 boneless, skinless chicken breasts
- 2 tablespoons fresh lemon juice
- 2 teaspoons dried oregano
- 1 teaspoon dried thyme
- Salt and pepper to taste

PreparationTime: 10 minutes
Cook Time: 30 minutes
Total Time: 40 minutes
Serves: 4 servings

Instructions:

1. Preheat your oven to 400°F (200°C).

2. Place the chicken breasts in a baking dish or on a rimmed baking sheet.

3. Drizzle the lemon juice over the chicken, making sure to coat all the pieces.

4. Sprinkle the dried oregano and thyme evenly over the chicken.

5. Season with salt and pepper to taste.

6. Bake the chicken for 25-30 minutes, or until it's cooked through and the juices run clear.

7. Serve the lemon herb chicken immediately, garnished with fresh lemon slices or chopped parsley if desired.

This recipe is perfect for those following a diabetic diet as it's low in carbs, high in protein, and uses simple, wholesome ingredients. The lemon and herbs add a delicious flavor without the need for any added sugars or sauces. Enjoy this easy and healthy Lemon Herb Chicken!

32. Baked Salmon

Ingredients:

- 4 (6 oz) salmon fillets
- 2 tablespoons olive oil
- 1 teaspoon garlic powder
- 1 teaspoon dried dill
- Salt and pepper to taste

PreparationTime: 5 minutes
Cook Time: 15 minutes
Total Time: 20 minutes
Serves: 4 servings

Instructions:

1. Preheat your oven to 400°F (200°C).

2. Line a baking sheet with parchment paper or foil.

3. Place the salmon fillets on the prepared baking sheet.

4. Drizzle the olive oil over the salmon, making sure to coat all the pieces.

5. Sprinkle the garlic powder and dried dill evenly over the salmon.

6. Season with salt and pepper to taste.

7. Bake the salmon for 12-15 minutes, or until it's cooked through and flakes easily with a fork.

8. Serve the baked salmon immediately, garnished with fresh lemon wedges or chopped parsley if desired.

This recipe is perfect for those following a diabetic diet as it's low in carbs, high in protein, and uses simple, wholesome ingredients. The olive oil, garlic, and dill add a delicious flavor without the need for any added sugars or sauces. Enjoy this easy and healthy Baked Salmon!

33. Beef Stir-Fry

Ingredients:

- 1 lb beef sirloin, thinly sliced
- 2 tablespoons low-sodium soy sauce
- 1 tablespoon rice vinegar
- 2 teaspoons sesame oil
- Salt and pepper to taste

PreparationTime: 10 minutes
Cook Time: 15 minutes
Total Time: 25 minutes
Serves: 4 servings

Instructions:

1. In a large skillet or wok, heat 1 tablespoon of sesame oil over high heat.

2. Add the sliced beef to the hot pan and stir-fry for 3-4 minutes, or until the beef is browned and cooked through. Transfer the beef to a plate and set aside.

3. In the same pan, add the remaining 1 tablespoon of sesame oil.

4. Add the soy sauce and rice vinegar to the pan and stir to combine.

5. Return the cooked beef to the pan and toss to coat the beef in the sauce.

6. Cook for an additional 2-3 minutes, or until the sauce has thickened slightly.

7. Season with salt and pepper to taste.

8. Serve the beef stir-fry immediately, over steamed cauliflower rice or zucchini noodles for a low-carb option.

This recipe is perfect for those following a diabetic diet as it's low in carbs, high in protein, and uses simple, wholesome ingredients. The soy sauce, rice vinegar, and sesame oil add a delicious flavor without the need for any added sugars or sauces. Enjoy this easy and healthy Beef Stir-Fry!

34. Stuffed Bell Peppers

Ingredients:

- 4 large bell peppers (any color)
- 1 lb ground turkey or lean ground beef
- 1 cup cooked brown rice
- 1 small onion, diced
- 2 cloves garlic, minced
- 1 (14.5 oz) can diced tomatoes
- 1 tsp dried oregano
- 1 tsp dried basil
- 1/2 tsp salt
- 1/4 tsp black pepper
- 1 cup shredded mozzarella cheese

PreparationTime: 20 minutes
Cook Time: 45 minutes
Total Time: 1 hour 5 minutes
Serves: 4 servings

Instructions:

1. Preheat your oven to 375°F (190°C).

2. Cut the tops off the bell peppers and remove the seeds and membranes. Place the peppers in a baking dish.

3. In a large skillet, cook the ground turkey or beef over medium heat until browned and crumbled, 5-7 minutes. Drain any excess fat.

4. Add the onion and garlic to the skillet and cook for 2-3 minutes until softened.

5. Stir in the cooked rice, diced tomatoes, oregano, basil, salt, and pepper. Mix well.

6. Spoon the filling mixture into the hollowed-out bell peppers, packing it in tightly.

7. Top each stuffed pepper with shredded mozzarella cheese.

8. Bake for 35-45 minutes, or until the peppers are tender and the cheese is melted and bubbly.

9. Serve the stuffed bell peppers hot, garnished with fresh parsley or basil if desired.

These Stuffed Bell Peppers are a delicious and healthy meal that's perfect for a weeknight dinner. The combination of ground meat, rice, and vegetables makes for a satisfying and nutritious dish.

35. Zucchini Noodles with Pesto

Ingredients:

- 4 medium zucchini, spiralized or julienned into noodles
- 1/2 cup basil pesto (store-bought or homemade)
- 2 tablespoons pine nuts (or chopped walnuts)
- 1/4 cup grated Parmesan cheese

PreparationTime: 10 minutes
Cook Time: 10 minutes
Total Time: 20 minutes
Serves: 4 servings

Instructions:

1. In a large skillet or wok, heat a small amount of olive oil or cooking spray over medium-high heat.

2. Add the zucchini noodles to the hot pan and sauté for 5-7 minutes, or until the noodles are tender but still have a slight bite.

3. Remove the pan from the heat and add the basil pesto. Toss the noodles to coat them evenly with the pesto.

4. Sprinkle the pine nuts (or walnuts) and grated Parmesan cheese over the top of the zucchini noodles.

5. Serve the Zucchini Noodles with Pesto immediately, while hot.

This recipe is perfect for those following a diabetic diet as it's low in carbs, high in fiber, and uses simple, wholesome ingredients. The zucchini noodles provide a delicious and nutritious alternative to traditional pasta, while the pesto, pine nuts, and Parmesan add a flavorful and satisfying touch. Enjoy this easy and healthy Zucchini Noodles with Pesto!

36. Grilled Chicken Breast

Ingredients:

- 4 (6 oz) boneless, skinless chicken breasts
- 2 tablespoons olive oil
- 1 teaspoon garlic powder
- 1 teaspoon dried Italian seasoning
- Salt and pepper to taste

PreparationTime: 5 minutes
Cook Time: 15 minutes
Total Time: 20 minutes
Serves: 4 servings

Instructions:

1. Preheat your grill or grill pan to medium-high heat.

2. Pat the chicken breasts dry with paper towels and place them in a shallow dish or resealable bag.

3. Drizzle the olive oil over the chicken and turn to coat both sides.

4. Sprinkle the garlic powder and dried Italian seasoning evenly over the chicken, rubbing it in to coat the surfaces.

5. Season the chicken with salt and pepper to taste.

6. Grill the chicken for 6-8 minutes per side, or until it's cooked through and the juices run clear.

7. Transfer the grilled chicken breasts to a clean plate and let them rest for 5 minutes before serving.

8. Serve the Grilled Chicken Breast immediately, garnished with fresh herbs or a squeeze of lemon if desired.

This recipe is perfect for those following a diabetic diet as it's low in carbs, high in protein, and uses simple, wholesome ingredients. The olive oil, garlic, and Italian seasoning add a delicious flavor without the need for any added sugars or sauces. Enjoy this easy and healthy Grilled Chicken Breast!

37. Pork Tenderloin with Apples

Ingredients:

Main Dishes

- 1 lb pork tenderloin, cut into 1-inch thick slices
- 2 medium apples, cored and sliced
- 2 tablespoons apple cider vinegar
- 1 teaspoon ground cinnamon
- Salt and pepper to taste

PreparationTime: 10 minutes
Cook Time: 25 minutes
Total Time: 35 minutes
Serves: 4 servings

Instructions:

1. Preheat your oven to 400°F (200°C).

2. Season the pork tenderloin slices with salt and pepper.

3. In a large oven-safe skillet or baking dish, arrange the pork tenderloin slices in a single layer.

4. Arrange the apple slices around and on top of the pork.

5. Drizzle the apple cider vinegar over the pork and apples.

6. Sprinkle the ground cinnamon evenly over the top.

7. Bake for 20-25 minutes, or until the pork is cooked through and the apples are tender.

8. Serve the Pork Tenderloin with Apples immediately, garnished with fresh parsley or thyme if desired.

This recipe is perfect for those following a diabetic diet as it's low in carbs, high in protein, and uses simple, wholesome ingredients. The apples and cinnamon add a delicious sweetness without the need for any added sugars. Enjoy this easy and healthy Pork Tenderloin with Apples!

38. Shrimp Scampi

Ingredients:

- 1 lb large shrimp, peeled and deveined
- 3 tablespoons unsalted butter
- 2 tablespoons lemon juice
- 2 cloves garlic, minced
- Salt and pepper to taste

PreparationTime: 10 minutes
Cook Time: 15 minutes
Total Time: 25 minutes
Serves: 4 servings

Instructions:

1. In a large skillet, melt the butter over medium heat.

2. Add the minced garlic to the melted butter and cook for 1-2 minutes, until fragrant.

3. Add the shrimp to the skillet and cook for 3-4 minutes, stirring occasionally, until the shrimp start to turn pink.

4. Squeeze the lemon juice over the shrimp and continue cooking for another 2-3 minutes, until the shrimp are fully cooked and opaque.

5. Season the shrimp scampi with salt and pepper to taste.

6. Serve the Shrimp Scampi immediately, over zucchini noodles or cauliflower rice for a low-carb option.

This recipe is perfect for those following a diabetic diet as it's low in carbs, high in protein, and uses simple, wholesome ingredients. The butter, lemon, and garlic add a delicious flavor without the need for any added sugars or sauces. Enjoy this easy and healthy Shrimp Scampi!

39. Turkey Meatballs

Ingredients:

Main Dishes

- 1 lb ground turkey
- 1/4 cup grated Parmesan cheese
- 2 tablespoons chopped fresh parsley
- 1 teaspoon garlic powder
- Salt and pepper to taste

PreparationTime: 15 minutes
Cook Time: 20 minutes
Total Time: 35 minutes
Serves: 4 servings (12 meatballs)

Instructions:

1. Preheat your oven to 400°F (200°C).

2. In a large bowl, combine the ground turkey, Parmesan cheese, parsley, and garlic powder. Mix well until the ingredients are evenly distributed.

3. Season the turkey mixture with salt and pepper to taste.

4. Using your hands, form the mixture into 12 equal-sized meatballs, about 1-1/2 inches in diameter.

5. Place the meatballs on a baking sheet lined with parchment paper or a silicone baking mat.

6. Bake the meatballs for 18-20 minutes, or until they are cooked through and no longer pink in the center.

7. Serve the Turkey Meatballs hot, either on their own or with a side of roasted vegetables or a salad.

This recipe is perfect for those following a diabetic diet as it's low in carbs, high in protein, and uses simple, wholesome ingredients. The Parmesan cheese and parsley add flavor without the need for any added sugars or sauces. Enjoy these easy and healthy Turkey Meatballs!

40. Garlic Butter Steak Bites

Ingredients:

- 1 lb sirloin steak, cut into 1-inch cubes
- 2 tbsp olive oil
- 3 cloves garlic, minced
- 4 tbsp unsalted butter, softened
- 2 tsp chopped fresh parsley
- 1/2 tsp salt
- 1/4 tsp black pepper

PreparationTime: 10 minutes
Cook Time: 10 minutes
Total Time: 20 minutes
Serves: 4

Instructions:

1. In a small bowl, mix together the softened butter, garlic, parsley, salt, and pepper until well combined. Set aside.

2. Heat the olive oil in a large skillet over high heat.

3. Working in batches if needed, add the steak cubes in a single layer and cook for 2-3 minutes per side, until nicely browned on the outside but still pink in the center.

4. Remove the steak bites from the skillet and transfer to a plate.

5. Immediately top the hot steak bites with the garlic butter mixture and toss to coat.

6. Serve the garlic butter steak bites immediately, while hot. Enjoy!

The key is to cook the steak bites quickly over high heat to get a nice sear on the outside while keeping the inside tender and juicy. The garlic butter melts right over the hot steak for maximum flavor.

41. Herb-Crusted Cod

Ingredients:

- 4 (6 oz) cod fillets
- 1/2 cup panko breadcrumbs
- 2 tbsp grated Parmesan cheese
- 2 tbsp chopped fresh parsley
- 1 tbsp chopped fresh thyme
- 1 tbsp chopped fresh rosemary
- 2 tsp lemon zest
- 1/4 tsp salt
- 1/4 tsp black pepper
- 2 tbsp olive oil

PreparationTime: 10 minutes
Cook Time: 15 minutes
Total Time: 25 minutes
Serves: 4

Instructions:

1. Preheat the oven to 400°F. Line a baking sheet with parchment paper.

2. In a shallow bowl, mix together the panko, Parmesan, parsley, thyme, rosemary, lemon zest, salt, and pepper.

3. Drizzle the olive oil over the cod fillets and turn to coat both sides.

4. Gently press the herb-breadcrumb mixture onto the top of each cod fillet, pressing to adhere.

5. Place the coated cod fillets on the prepared baking sheet.

6. Bake for 12-15 minutes, until the cod is opaque and flakes easily with a fork and the topping is golden brown.

7. Serve the herb-crusted cod immediately, garnished with extra chopped parsley if desired.

The crispy, flavorful breadcrumb topping complements the tender, flaky cod perfectly in this easy baked fish dish. Enjoy!

42. Chicken Fajitas

Ingredients:

- 1 lb boneless, skinless chicken breasts, sliced into strips
- 1 large bell pepper, sliced into strips
- 1 large onion, sliced into strips
- 1 tbsp fajita seasoning (no-sugar added)

PreparationTime: 10 minutes
Cook Time: 15 minutes
Total Time: 25 minutes
Serves: 4

Instructions:

1. In a large skillet or wok, heat a small amount of cooking spray or olive oil over medium-high heat.

2. Add the sliced chicken, bell pepper, and onion to the hot pan. Sprinkle the fajita seasoning over the top.

3. Cook, stirring frequently, for 12-15 minutes until the chicken is cooked through and the vegetables are tender.

4. Serve the chicken fajita mixture warm, wrapped in low-carb tortillas or lettuce leaves. Top with any desired diabetic-friendly toppings like avocado, salsa, shredded cheese, etc.

Tips:
- Use a low-sodium fajita seasoning or make your own with spices like chili powder, cumin, garlic powder, and oregano.

- Pair with a side salad or roasted vegetables for a complete diabetic-friendly meal.

- This recipe is also gluten-free if you use gluten-free tortillas or lettuce wraps.

The simple combination of chicken, peppers, and onions seasoned with a flavorful fajita spice mix makes this a quick and easy diabetic-friendly dinner option.

43. Balsamic Glazed Pork Chops

Ingredients:

Main Dishes

- 4 (4-6 oz) boneless pork chops
- 1/4 cup balsamic vinegar
- 2 tbsp Dijon mustard
- 1 tbsp sugar-free maple syrup or honey

PreparationTime: 5 minutes
Cook Time: 15 minutes
Total Time: 20 minutes
Serves: 4

Instructions:

1. Preheat your oven to 400°F.

2. In a small bowl, whisk together the balsamic vinegar, Dijon mustard, and maple syrup/honey.

3. Place the pork chops in a baking dish or on a rimmed baking sheet. Pour the balsamic glaze over the top, making sure to coat the chops evenly.

4. Bake for 12-15 minutes, flipping the chops halfway through, until the pork is cooked through and reaches an internal temperature of 145°F.

5. Remove the pork chops from the oven and let rest for 3-5 minutes.

6. Serve the balsamic glazed pork chops warm, spooning any extra glaze from the pan over the top.

Tips:
- Pair with roasted vegetables or a fresh salad for a complete diabetic-friendly meal.
- The balsamic glaze provides a sweet and tangy flavor without a lot of added sugar.
- You can also grill the pork chops instead of baking them.

This simple 4-ingredient recipe results in tender, flavorful pork chops that are perfect for a diabetic-friendly dinner.

44. Honey Mustard Chicken

Ingredients:

- 4 (6 oz) boneless, skinless chicken breasts
- 2 tbsp Dijon mustard
- 2 tbsp sugar-free honey or maple syrup
- 1 tsp dried thyme

PreparationTime: 5 minutes
Cook Time: 25 minutes
Total Time: 30 minutes
Serves: 4

Instructions:

1. Preheat your oven to 400°F. Lightly grease a baking dish or line a baking sheet with parchment paper.

2. In a small bowl, whisk together the Dijon mustard, sugar-free honey/maple syrup, and dried thyme.

3. Place the chicken breasts in the prepared baking dish or on the baking sheet. Spoon the honey mustard mixture evenly over the top of the chicken, making sure to coat all sides.

4. Bake for 20-25 minutes, until the chicken is cooked through and reaches an internal temperature of 165°F.

5. Remove the honey mustard chicken from the oven and let rest for 5 minutes before serving.

Tips:
- Serve the chicken with roasted vegetables or a fresh salad for a complete diabetic-friendly meal.
- You can also grill the chicken instead of baking it.
- For extra flavor, you can add a sprinkle of garlic powder or paprika to the honey mustard mixture.

This simple 4-ingredient recipe results in tender, flavorful chicken that is perfect for a diabetic-friendly dinner. The honey mustard glaze adds a delicious sweet and tangy flavor.

45. Tuna Salad Lettuce Wraps

Ingredients:

Main Dishes

- 2 (5 oz) cans tuna, drained and flaked
- 2 tbsp plain Greek yogurt
- 1 tbsp Dijon mustard
- 1/4 tsp black pepper
- 8 large lettuce leaves (such as romaine or butter lettuce)

PreparationTime: 10 minutes
Total Time: 10 minutes
Serves: 4

Instructions:

1. In a medium bowl, mix together the drained tuna, Greek yogurt, Dijon mustard, and black pepper until well combined.

2. Lay the lettuce leaves flat on a plate or cutting board. Scoop about 1/4 cup of the tuna salad mixture onto the center of each lettuce leaf.

3. Fold the sides of the lettuce leaf over the tuna salad and enjoy immediately.

Tips:
- For extra crunch, you can add diced celery, onion, or dill pickles to the tuna salad.

- Serve the tuna salad lettuce wraps with a side of sliced cucumber, cherry tomatoes, or a small salad.

- This recipe is also great for meal prep - make the tuna salad in advance and assemble the wraps when ready to eat.

This simple 4-ingredient tuna salad is a great diabetic-friendly option. The lettuce wraps provide a low-carb, high-fiber alternative to traditional bread or crackers. Enjoy this easy and nutritious lunch or snack!

46. Lemon Garlic Shrimp

Ingredients:

- 1 lb large shrimp, peeled and deveined
- 3 tbsp olive oil
- 4 cloves garlic, minced
- 1 tbsp lemon juice
- 2 tsp lemon zest
- 1/4 tsp red pepper flakes (optional)
- 1/4 cup chopped fresh parsley
- Salt and black pepper to taste

PreparationTime: 10 minutes
Cook Time: 10 minutes
Total Time: 20 minutes
Serves: 4

Instructions:

1. In a large skillet, heat the olive oil over medium-high heat.

2. Add the minced garlic and sauté for 1 minute, until fragrant.

3. Add the shrimp to the skillet and cook for 2-3 minutes per side, until the shrimp are pink and opaque.

4. Stir in the lemon juice, lemon zest, and red pepper flakes (if using). Cook for 1 more minute.

5. Remove the skillet from heat and stir in the chopped parsley. Season with salt and black pepper to taste.

6. Serve the lemon garlic shrimp immediately, while hot. Enjoy!

Tips:
- Serve the shrimp over pasta, rice, or with a side salad for a complete meal.
- For extra flavor, you can add a splash of white wine or chicken broth to the skillet.
- Adjust the amount of red pepper flakes to your desired level of spiciness.

The bright lemon and garlic flavors pair perfectly with the tender, juicy shrimp in this easy and flavorful dish. It's a quick and delicious option for a weeknight dinner.

47. Beef and Broccoli

Ingredients:

- 1 lb flank steak, thinly sliced against the grain
- 2 tbsp soy sauce
- 1 tbsp rice vinegar
- 1 tbsp brown sugar
- 2 tsp sesame oil
- 2 cloves garlic, minced
- 1 tsp grated fresh ginger
- 2 tbsp vegetable oil
- 4 cups broccoli florets
- 2 green onions, sliced
- Sesame seeds for garnish (optional)

PreparationTime: 15 minutes
Cook Time: 15 minutes
Total Time: 30 minutes
Serves: 4

Instructions:

1. In a medium bowl, combine the sliced flank steak, soy sauce, rice vinegar, brown sugar, sesame oil, garlic, and ginger. Toss to coat the beef and let marinate for 10-15 minutes.

2. Heat the vegetable oil in a large skillet or wok over high heat.

3. Add the marinated beef and stir-fry for 2-3 minutes until the beef is mostly cooked through.

4. Add the broccoli florets to the skillet and continue to stir-fry for 3-4 minutes, until the broccoli is tender-crisp.

5. Remove the skillet from heat and stir in the sliced green onions.

6. Serve the beef and broccoli immediately, garnished with sesame seeds if desired. Enjoy!

Tips:
- Serve over steamed rice or noodles for a complete meal.
- For extra flavor, you can add a splash of Worcestershire sauce or oyster sauce to the marinade.
- Adjust the cooking time for the broccoli based on your desired level of doneness.

This classic beef and broccoli stir-fry is quick, easy, and full of savory Asian-inspired flavors. It's a great weeknight dinner option.

48. Chicken Parmesan

Ingredients:

Main Dishes

- 4 boneless, skinless chicken breasts
- 1/2 cup all-purpose flour
- 2 eggs, beaten
- 1 cup panko breadcrumbs
- 1/2 cup grated Parmesan cheese
- 1 tsp dried oregano
- 1/2 tsp garlic powder
- 1/4 tsp salt
- 1/4 tsp black pepper
- 2 tbsp olive oil
- 1 jar (24 oz) marinara sauce
- 1 cup shredded mozzarella cheese

PreparationTime: 20 minutes
Cook Time: 30 minutes
Total Time: 50 minutes
Serves: 4

Instructions:

1. Preheat your oven to 400°F. Lightly grease a baking dish or line a baking sheet with parchment paper.

2. Set up a breading station with three shallow dishes: one with the flour, one with the beaten eggs, and one with the panko breadcrumbs, Parmesan, oregano, garlic powder, salt, and pepper mixed together.

3. Dredge each chicken breast in the flour, dip in the egg, and then coat in the breadcrumb mixture, pressing to adhere.

4. Heat the olive oil in a large skillet over medium-high heat. Working in batches if needed, add the breaded chicken and cook for 2-3 minutes per side until golden brown.

5. Transfer the partially cooked chicken to the prepared baking dish or sheet. Top each chicken breast with about 1/4 cup of the marinara sauce and sprinkle with the shredded mozzarella cheese.

6. Bake for 15-20 minutes, until the chicken is cooked through and the cheese is melted and bubbly. Serve the chicken parmesan hot, garnished with fresh basil or parsley if desired. Enjoy!

This classic chicken parmesan dish features crispy, breaded chicken breasts topped with marinara sauce and melted mozzarella cheese. It's a family-friendly dinner that's sure to please.

49. BBQ Pulled Chicken

Ingredients:

- 2 lbs boneless, skinless chicken breasts
- 1 cup no-sugar-added BBQ sauce
- 1 tbsp Dijon mustard
- 1 tsp garlic powder

PreparationTime: 5 minutes
Cook Time: 4-6 hours
Total Time: 4-6 hours 5 minutes
Serves: 4-6

Instructions:

1. Place the chicken breasts in a slow cooker.

2. In a small bowl, whisk together the BBQ sauce, Dijon mustard, and garlic powder. Pour the sauce over the chicken, making sure the chicken is well coated.

3. Cover the slow cooker and cook on low for 4-6 hours, until the chicken is very tender and shreds easily with a fork.

4. Remove the chicken from the slow cooker and shred it using two forks. Return the shredded chicken to the slow cooker and toss it with the remaining sauce.

5. Serve the BBQ pulled chicken warm, over a bed of cauliflower rice, on a lettuce wrap, or with a side salad for a complete diabetic-friendly meal.

Tips:
- Use a no-sugar-added or low-sugar BBQ sauce to keep this recipe diabetic-friendly.
- For extra flavor, you can add a pinch of smoked paprika or chili powder to the sauce.
- This pulled chicken also makes a great topping for baked potatoes or as a filling for lettuce wraps.

This simple 4-ingredient BBQ pulled chicken is perfect for a diabetic-friendly dinner. The slow cooker makes it easy to prepare, and the flavorful sauce keeps the chicken moist and delicious.

50. Teriyaki Salmon

Ingredients:

- 4 (6 oz) salmon fillets
- 1/4 cup no-sugar-added teriyaki sauce
- 1 tbsp rice vinegar
- 1 tsp sesame oil

Main Dishes

PreparationTime: 5 minutes
Cook Time: 12 minutes
Total Time: 17 minutes
Serves: 4

Instructions:

1. Preheat your oven to 400°F. Line a baking sheet with parchment paper or foil.

2. Place the salmon fillets skin-side down on the prepared baking sheet.

3. In a small bowl, whisk together the teriyaki sauce, rice vinegar, and sesame oil.

4. Spoon the teriyaki sauce mixture evenly over the top of the salmon fillets, making sure to coat them completely.

5. Bake for 10-12 minutes, until the salmon is cooked through and flakes easily with a fork.

6. Serve the teriyaki salmon immediately, garnished with sliced green onions or sesame seeds if desired.

Tips:
- Pair the salmon with steamed broccoli or a fresh salad for a complete diabetic-friendly meal.

- For extra flavor, you can add a sprinkle of garlic powder or grated ginger to the teriyaki sauce.

- This recipe also works well with other types of fish, such as tilapia or halibut.

The simple teriyaki glaze adds a delicious sweet and savory flavor to the tender, flaky salmon. This 4-ingredient dish is a quick and easy diabetic-friendly option for a weeknight dinner.

51. Chickpea Curry

Ingredients:

- 2 (15 oz) cans chickpeas, drained and rinsed
- 1 (14 oz) can diced tomatoes
- 1 cup light coconut milk
- 2 tbsp curry powder

PreparationTime: 10 minutes
Cook Time: 20 minutes
Total Time: 30 minutes
Serves: 4

Instructions:

1. In a large skillet or saucepan, combine the drained and rinsed chickpeas, diced tomatoes, coconut milk, and curry powder.

2. Bring the mixture to a simmer over medium heat, stirring occasionally.

3. Reduce the heat to low and let the curry simmer for 15-20 minutes, until the flavors have melded and the sauce has thickened slightly.

4. Serve the chickpea curry warm, over a bed of cauliflower rice or with a side of roasted vegetables for a complete diabetic-friendly meal.

Tips:
- Use a mild or medium curry powder to control the spice level. Adjust the amount to your taste preferences.

- For extra flavor, you can add a pinch of cumin, grated ginger, or chopped fresh cilantro.

- This recipe is also vegan and gluten-free, making it a great option for those with dietary restrictions.

The combination of protein-packed chickpeas, tangy tomatoes, and creamy coconut milk creates a delicious and satisfying curry that is perfect for a diabetic-friendly dinner. It's quick, easy, and full of flavor!

52. Black Bean Tacos

Ingredients:

- 1 (15 oz) can black beans, drained and rinsed
- 1 tsp ground cumin
- 1/4 tsp chili powder
- 8 small low-carb tortillas or lettuce leaves

PreparationTime: 10 minutes
Cook Time: 10 minutes
Total Time: 20 minutes
Serves: 4

Instructions:

1. In a medium saucepan, combine the drained and rinsed black beans, ground cumin, and chili powder.

2. Heat the black bean mixture over medium heat, stirring occasionally, until heated through, about 5-7 minutes.

3. Using a fork or potato masher, lightly mash the black beans, leaving some whole beans intact.

4. Spoon the seasoned black bean mixture into the low-carb tortillas or lettuce leaves.

5. Top the black bean tacos with your desired diabetic-friendly toppings, such as diced avocado, shredded lettuce, salsa, or a sprinkle of low-fat shredded cheese.

6. Serve the black bean tacos immediately and enjoy!

Tips:
- For extra flavor, you can add a minced garlic clove or a squeeze of fresh lime juice to the black bean mixture.

- Serve the black bean tacos with a side of roasted vegetables or a fresh salad for a complete diabetic-friendly meal.

- This recipe is also gluten-free if you use lettuce leaves instead of tortillas.

These simple 4-ingredient black bean tacos are a quick, easy, and diabetic-friendly option for a weeknight dinner or lunch. The flavorful black beans are the star of the show!

53. Vegetable Stir-Fry

Ingredients:

- 2 cups mixed fresh vegetables
(such as broccoli, bell peppers, snap peas,
 and mushrooms),
chopped into bite-sized pieces
- 2 tbsp low-sodium soy sauce
- 1 tbsp rice vinegar
- 1 tsp sesame oil

PreparationTime: 10 minutes
Cook Time: 15 minutes
Total Time: 25 minutes
Serves: 4

Instructions:

1. Heat a large skillet or wok over high heat. Add the chopped vegetables and stir-fry for 5-7 minutes, until they are tender-crisp.

2. In a small bowl, whisk together the soy sauce, rice vinegar, and sesame oil.

3. Add the sauce mixture to the skillet with the vegetables and toss to coat everything evenly.

4. Continue to stir-fry for 2-3 minutes, until the sauce has thickened slightly.

5. Serve the vegetable stir-fry immediately, over a bed of cauliflower rice or steamed brown rice if desired.

Tips:
- Use a variety of fresh, colorful vegetables to get a range of nutrients.
- Adjust the cooking time for the vegetables based on your desired level of doneness.
- For extra protein, you can add cooked chicken, shrimp, or tofu to the stir-fry.
- Garnish with sliced green onions, sesame seeds, or a sprinkle of crushed red pepper flakes.

This simple 4-ingredient vegetable stir-fry is a quick, easy, and diabetic-friendly way to get in a serving of healthy veggies. The flavorful sauce ties everything together for a delicious and nutritious meal.

54. Lentil Salad

Ingredients:

- 1 (15 oz) can lentils, drained and rinsed
- 1/2 cup diced cucumber
- 2 tbsp red wine vinegar
- 1 tsp Dijon mustard

PreparationTime: 10 minutes
Chill Time: 30 minutes
Total Time: 40 minutes
Serves: 4

Instructions:

1. In a medium bowl, combine the drained and rinsed lentils, diced cucumber, red wine vinegar, and Dijon mustard.

2. Stir everything together until well mixed.

3. Cover the bowl and refrigerate the lentil salad for at least 30 minutes to allow the flavors to meld.

4. Serve the chilled lentil salad as a side dish or light main course. It pairs well with grilled chicken, fish, or roasted vegetables.

Tips:
- For extra flavor, you can add a pinch of dried oregano, basil, or garlic powder to the salad.

- Swap the cucumber for other diced veggies like bell peppers, tomatoes, or onions.

- This lentil salad is a great make-ahead option - it will keep well in the refrigerator for 3-4 days.

- To make it a more substantial meal, you can add cooked quinoa, chickpeas, or chopped nuts.

This simple 4-ingredient lentil salad is a delicious and diabetic-friendly option for a light lunch or side dish. The tangy vinaigrette dressing complements the earthy lentils and crisp vegetables perfectly.

55. Tofu Scramble

Ingredients:

- 1 (14 oz) block extra-firm tofu,
drained and crumbled
- 2 tbsp nutritional yeast
- 1 tsp turmeric
- 1/4 tsp salt

PreparationTime: 5 minutes
Cook Time: 10 minutes
Total Time: 15 minutes
Serves: 4

Instructions:

1. In a large skillet over medium heat, crumble the drained tofu into small pieces.

2. Add the nutritional yeast, turmeric, and salt to the skillet. Stir everything together until the tofu is well coated with the spices.

3. Continue to cook the tofu scramble, stirring occasionally, for 8-10 minutes, until the tofu is heated through and has a slightly dry, scrambled texture.

4. Serve the tofu scramble warm, on its own or with your choice of diabetic-friendly toppings such as diced avocado, salsa, or sautéed spinach.

Tips:
- For extra flavor, you can add minced garlic, diced onions, or chopped bell peppers to the scramble.

- Swap the nutritional yeast for a sprinkle of grated Parmesan cheese if desired.

- This tofu scramble is a great source of plant-based protein and can be enjoyed for breakfast, lunch, or dinner.

- Pair it with a side of roasted potatoes or a fresh salad for a complete diabetic-friendly meal.

This simple 4-ingredient tofu scramble is a quick, easy, and nutritious option for those following a diabetic diet. The turmeric and nutritional yeast give it a delicious, egg-like flavor and texture.

56. Quinoa and Black Bean Salad

Ingredients:

- 1 cup cooked quinoa, cooled
- 1 (15 oz) can black beans, drained and rinsed
- 1/2 cup diced cucumber
- 2 tbsp lime juice

PreparationTime: 10 minutes
Chill Time: 30 minutes
Total Time: 40 minutes
Serves: 4

Instructions:

1. In a medium bowl, combine the cooked and cooled quinoa, drained and rinsed black beans, and diced cucumber.

2. Drizzle the lime juice over the salad and gently toss everything together until well mixed.

3. Cover the bowl and refrigerate the quinoa and black bean salad for at least 30 minutes to allow the flavors to meld.

4. Serve the chilled salad as a side dish or light main course. It pairs well with grilled chicken, fish, or roasted vegetables.

Tips:
- For extra flavor, you can add a pinch of cumin, chili powder, or chopped fresh cilantro to the salad.

- Swap the cucumber for other diced veggies like bell peppers, tomatoes, or red onion.

- This salad is a great make-ahead option - it will keep well in the refrigerator for 3-4 days.

- To make it a more substantial meal, you can add cooked chicken, shrimp, or crumbled feta cheese.

This simple 4-ingredient quinoa and black bean salad is a delicious and diabetic-friendly option for a light lunch or side dish. The bright lime dressing complements the nutty quinoa and protein-packed black beans perfectly.

57. Cauliflower Fried Rice

Ingredients:

- 1 head of cauliflower, riced
(about 4 cups riced cauliflower)
- 1 cup frozen peas and carrots
- 2 tbsp low-sodium soy sauce
- 2 eggs, lightly beaten

PreparationTime: 10 minutes
Cook Time: 15 minutes
Total Time: 25 minutes
Serves: 4

Instructions:

1. In a large skillet or wok, heat a small amount of cooking spray or olive oil over medium-high heat.

2. Add the riced cauliflower and frozen peas and carrots to the skillet. Stir-fry for 5-7 minutes, until the vegetables are tender.

3. Push the vegetables to the side of the skillet and pour the beaten eggs into the empty space. Scramble the eggs, then mix them into the vegetable mixture.

4. Drizzle the soy sauce over the cauliflower fried rice and stir everything together until well combined.

5. Serve the cauliflower fried rice warm, as a main dish or side.

Tips:
- For extra flavor, you can add minced garlic, grated ginger, or chopped green onions to the fried rice.

- Customize the vegetables by using other frozen or fresh options like broccoli, bell peppers, or mushrooms.

- This recipe is also great for meal prep - the fried rice will keep well in the refrigerator for 3-4 days.

- To make it a more substantial meal, you can add cooked chicken, shrimp, or tofu to the fried rice.

This simple 4-ingredient cauliflower fried rice is a delicious and diabetic-friendly alternative to traditional fried rice. It's a quick and easy way to get in a serving of low-carb veggies.

58. Sweet Potato and Black Bean Chili

Ingredients:

- 1 (15 oz) can black beans, drained and rinsed
- 1 (15 oz) can diced tomatoes
- 1 medium sweet potato, peeled and diced
- 2 tbsp chili powder

PreparationTime: 10 minutes
Cook Time: 30 minutes
Total Time: 40 minutes
Serves: 4

Instructions:

1. In a large pot or Dutch oven, combine the drained and rinsed black beans, diced tomatoes, diced sweet potato, and chili powder.

2. Bring the mixture to a boil over medium-high heat, then reduce the heat to low and let the chili simmer for 25-30 minutes, stirring occasionally, until the sweet potato is tender.

3. Taste the chili and adjust the seasoning with additional chili powder, salt, or pepper as needed.

4. Serve the sweet potato and black bean chili warm, garnished with diced avocado, chopped cilantro, or a sprinkle of low-fat shredded cheese if desired.

Tips:
- For extra flavor, you can add minced garlic, diced onion, or a pinch of cumin to the chili.

- Adjust the amount of chili powder to control the spice level, depending on your preferences.

- This chili is a great make-ahead option - it will keep well in the refrigerator for 3-4 days or can be frozen for longer storage.

- Serve the chili over a bed of cauliflower rice or with a side salad for a complete diabetic-friendly meal.

The sweet potato and black beans in this simple 4-ingredient chili provide a delicious and nutritious combination of complex carbohydrates, fiber, and protein. It's a comforting and diabetic-friendly dish that's perfect for a weeknight dinner.

59. Roasted Vegetable Medley

Ingredients:

- 1 lb mixed vegetables
(such as broccoli, cauliflower,
Brussels sprouts, and carrots),
cut into bite-sized pieces
- 2 tbsp olive oil
- 1 tsp dried Italian seasoning
- 1/4 tsp salt

PreparationTime: 10 minutes
Cook Time: 25 minutes
Total Time: 35 minutes
Serves: 4

Instructions:

1. Preheat your oven to 400°F. Line a large baking sheet with parchment paper.

2. In a large bowl, toss the cut vegetables with the olive oil, Italian seasoning, and salt until the vegetables are evenly coated.

3. Spread the seasoned vegetables in a single layer on the prepared baking sheet.

4. Roast the vegetables for 20-25 minutes, stirring halfway, until they are tender and lightly browned.

5. Serve the roasted vegetable medley warm, as a side dish or main course. Garnish with a sprinkle of grated Parmesan cheese or chopped fresh herbs if desired.

Tips:
- Use a variety of colorful vegetables to get a range of nutrients and flavors.

- Adjust the roasting time based on the size and density of the vegetables you're using.

- For extra flavor, you can add minced garlic, lemon zest, or a drizzle of balsamic glaze to the vegetables.

- This recipe is also great for meal prep - the roasted veggies will keep well in the refrigerator for 3-4 days.

This simple 4-ingredient roasted vegetable medley is a delicious and diabetic-friendly way to enjoy a variety of nutrient-dense vegetables. It's a versatile side dish that pairs well with grilled proteins or can be the star of a meatless main course.

60. Stuffed Portobello Mushrooms

Ingredients:

- 4 large portobello mushroom caps,
 stems removed and chopped
- 1 cup crumbled feta cheese
- 1/4 cup chopped fresh spinach
- 1 tbsp olive oil

PreparationTime: 10 minutes
Cook Time: 20 minutes
Total Time: 30 minutes
Serves: 4

Instructions:

1. Preheat your oven to 400°F. Line a baking sheet with parchment paper.

2. Gently clean the portobello mushroom caps with a damp paper towel. Remove and chop the stems.

3. In a small bowl, mix together the chopped mushroom stems, crumbled feta cheese, and chopped spinach.

4. Brush the outside of the mushroom caps with the olive oil and place them cap-side up on the prepared baking sheet.

5. Spoon the feta and spinach mixture evenly into the mushroom caps, packing it down gently.

6. Bake the stuffed portobello mushrooms for 15-20 minutes, until the mushrooms are tender and the filling is hot and bubbly.

7. Serve the stuffed portobello mushrooms warm, as a main dish or appetizer.

Tips:
- For extra flavor, you can add a sprinkle of garlic powder, dried oregano, or red pepper flakes to the filling.
- Swap the feta cheese for shredded mozzarella or crumbled goat cheese if desired.
- Serve the stuffed mushrooms over a bed of mixed greens or with a side salad for a complete diabetic-friendly meal.
- This recipe is also great for meal prep - the baked stuffed mushrooms will keep well in the refrigerator for 3-4 days.

These simple 4-ingredient stuffed portobello mushrooms are a delicious and diabetic-friendly option for a quick and easy dinner or appetizer. The savory feta and spinach filling complements the meaty mushroom caps perfectly.

61. Veggie Burger Patties

Ingredients:

- 1 (15 oz) can black beans, drained and rinsed
- 1 cup cooked quinoa
- 1/4 cup rolled oats
- 1 tsp garlic powder

PreparationTime: 15 minutes
Cook Time: 10 minutes
Total Time: 25 minutes
Serves: 4 (makes 4 patties)

Instructions:

1. In a large bowl, mash the drained and rinsed black beans with a fork or potato masher until they are mostly smooth with some whole beans remaining.

2. Add the cooked quinoa, rolled oats, and garlic powder to the mashed black beans. Stir everything together until well combined.

3. Divide the black bean and quinoa mixture into 4 equal portions and shape them into patty forms, about 1/2 inch thick.

4. Heat a large skillet or grill pan over medium heat. Cook the veggie burger patties for 4-5 minutes per side, until they are lightly browned and heated through.

5. Serve the veggie burger patties on a bed of lettuce, in a low-carb bun, or alongside your favorite diabetic-friendly toppings and sides.

Tips:
- For extra flavor, you can add diced onion, shredded carrot, or chopped fresh herbs to the patty mixture.

- These veggie burgers can be made ahead of time and refrigerated or frozen for later use.

- To freeze, place the uncooked patties on a baking sheet and freeze until firm, then transfer to an airtight container or resealable bag.

- When ready to cook, thaw the frozen patties and cook as directed.

These simple 4-ingredient veggie burger patties are a delicious and diabetic-friendly alternative to traditional beef burgers. The combination of black beans and quinoa provides a good source of plant-based protein and fiber.

62. Eggplant Parmesan

Ingredients:

- 1 medium eggplant, sliced into 1/2-inch thick rounds
- 1 cup marinara sauce
- 1 cup shredded part-skim mozzarella cheese
- 1/4 cup grated Parmesan cheese

PreparationTime: 15 minutes
Cook Time: 30 minutes
Total Time: 45 minutes
Serves: 4

Instructions:

1. Preheat your oven to 375°F. Lightly grease a 9x13 inch baking dish.

2. Arrange the eggplant slices in a single layer in the prepared baking dish.

3. Spoon the marinara sauce evenly over the eggplant slices, making sure to cover them completely.

4. Sprinkle the shredded mozzarella cheese and grated Parmesan cheese over the top of the sauce-covered eggplant.

5. Bake the eggplant parmesan for 25-30 minutes, until the eggplant is tender and the cheese is melted and bubbly.

6. Remove the eggplant parmesan from the oven and let it cool for 5 minutes before serving.

Tips:
- For extra flavor, you can add a sprinkle of dried oregano or basil to the top of the dish.
- Serve the eggplant parmesan over a bed of zucchini noodles or cauliflower rice for a low-carb meal.
- This dish can be made ahead of time and refrigerated or frozen for later use.
- To reheat, simply bake the eggplant parmesan in a preheated oven until heated through.

This simple 4-ingredient eggplant parmesan is a delicious and diabetic-friendly take on the classic Italian dish. The tender eggplant, tangy marinara sauce, and melted cheeses make for a satisfying and nutritious meal.

63. Spinach and Mushroom Quesadillas

Ingredients:

Vegetarian and Vegan Dishes

PreparationTime: 10 minutes
Cook Time: 10 minutes
Total Time: 20 minutes
Serves: 4

- 8 small low-carb tortillas or wraps
- 1 cup sliced mushrooms
- 1 cup fresh spinach leaves
- 1/2 cup shredded low-fat cheddar cheese

Instructions:

1. Heat a large skillet or griddle over medium heat.

2. Place 4 of the low-carb tortillas or wraps on the hot surface. Divide the sliced mushrooms and fresh spinach leaves evenly over the tortillas.

3. Sprinkle the shredded cheddar cheese over the mushrooms and spinach.

4. Top each quesadilla with the remaining 4 tortillas or wraps.

5. Cook the quesadillas for 2-3 minutes per side, until the tortillas are lightly browned and the cheese is melted.

6. Remove the quesadillas from the heat and cut each one into halves or quarters.

7. Serve the spinach and mushroom quesadillas warm, with a side of salsa, guacamole, or plain Greek yogurt for dipping.

Tips:
- For extra flavor, you can add a sprinkle of garlic powder, cumin, or chili powder to the filling.
- Swap the cheddar cheese for shredded mozzarella or pepper jack if desired.
- These quesadillas can be made ahead of time and reheated in the oven or microwave when ready to serve.
- Pair the quesadillas with a fresh salad or roasted vegetables for a complete diabetic-friendly meal.

These simple 4-ingredient spinach and mushroom quesadillas are a delicious and easy-to-make option for a diabetic-friendly lunch or dinner. The combination of nutrient-dense veggies and melted cheese makes for a satisfying and flavorful meal.

64. Broccoli and Cheese Stuffed Peppers

Ingredients:

- 4 medium bell peppers,
halved lengthwise and seeded
- 2 cups chopped broccoli florets
- 1 cup shredded low-fat cheddar cheese
- 1/4 cup water

PreparationTime: 15 minutes
Cook Time: 25 minutes
Total Time: 40 minutes
Serves: 4

Instructions:

1. Preheat your oven to 375°F. Lightly grease a baking dish or line it with parchment paper.

2. Arrange the bell pepper halves in the prepared baking dish, cut-side up.

3. In a medium bowl, mix together the chopped broccoli florets and shredded cheddar cheese.

4. Spoon the broccoli and cheese mixture evenly into the bell pepper halves, packing it down gently.

5. Pour the 1/4 cup of water into the bottom of the baking dish, around the stuffed peppers.

6. Cover the dish with foil and bake for 20-25 minutes, until the peppers are tender and the cheese is melted.

7. Remove the foil and broil the stuffed peppers for 2-3 minutes, until the cheese is lightly browned on top. Serve the broccoli and cheese stuffed peppers warm.

Tips:
- For extra flavor, you can add a sprinkle of garlic powder, dried oregano, or crushed red pepper flakes to the filling.
- Swap the cheddar cheese for shredded mozzarella or Parmesan if desired.
- Serve the stuffed peppers over a bed of cauliflower rice or with a side salad for a complete diabetic-friendly meal.
- This recipe can be made ahead of time and refrigerated or frozen for later use.

These simple 4-ingredient broccoli and cheese stuffed peppers are a delicious and diabetic-friendly way to enjoy a nutritious and satisfying meal. The combination of tender bell peppers, fresh broccoli, and melted cheese makes for a flavorful and filling dish.

65. Cauliflower Tacos

Ingredients:

- 1 head of cauliflower, cut into small florets
- 1 tbsp olive oil
- 1 tsp taco seasoning
- 8 small low-carb tortillas or lettuce leaves

PreparationTime: 10 minutes
Cook Time: 20 minutes
Total Time: 30 minutes
Serves: 4

Instructions:

1. Preheat your oven to 400°F. Line a baking sheet with parchment paper.

2. In a large bowl, toss the cauliflower florets with the olive oil and taco seasoning until the cauliflower is evenly coated.

3. Spread the seasoned cauliflower in a single layer on the prepared baking sheet.

4. Roast the cauliflower for 15-20 minutes, stirring halfway, until it is tender and lightly browned.

5. Remove the roasted cauliflower from the oven and let it cool slightly.

6. Divide the roasted cauliflower evenly among the low-carb tortillas or lettuce leaves.

7. Serve the cauliflower tacos immediately, with any desired diabetic-friendly toppings such as diced avocado, salsa, or plain Greek yogurt.

Tips:
- For extra flavor, you can add a pinch of cumin, chili powder, or garlic powder to the taco seasoning.
- Swap the low-carb tortillas for large lettuce leaves, such as romaine or butter lettuce, for a lower-carb option.
- These cauliflower tacos can be made ahead of time - the roasted cauliflower will keep well in the refrigerator for 3-4 days.
- Serve the cauliflower tacos with a side of roasted vegetables or a fresh salad for a complete diabetic-friendly meal.

These simple 4-ingredient cauliflower tacos are a delicious and diabetic-friendly alternative to traditional meat-based tacos. The roasted cauliflower provides a satisfying and nutritious filling for the low-carb tortillas or lettuce wraps.

66. Baked Falafel

Ingredients:

- 1 (15 oz) can chickpeas, drained and rinsed
- 2 tbsp whole wheat flour
- 1 tsp ground cumin
- 1/4 tsp salt

PreparationTime: 10 minutes
Cook Time: 20 minutes
Total Time: 30 minutes
Serves: 4 (makes 12 falafel)

Instructions:

1. Preheat your oven to 400°F. Line a baking sheet with parchment paper.

2. In a food processor, combine the drained and rinsed chickpeas, whole wheat flour, ground cumin, and salt. Pulse the mixture until it forms a coarse paste, but still has some texture.

3. Scoop the chickpea mixture by the tablespoonful and shape it into small patties or balls, about 1-inch in size.

4. Place the shaped falafel on the prepared baking sheet, spacing them apart.

5. Bake the falafel for 18-20 minutes, flipping them halfway through, until they are golden brown and crispy.

6. Serve the baked falafel warm, in pita bread or lettuce wraps, with your choice of diabetic-friendly toppings such as diced tomatoes, cucumber, red onion, and tahini sauce.

Tips:
- For extra flavor, you can add minced garlic, chopped fresh parsley, or a pinch of cayenne pepper to the falafel mixture.
- These baked falafel can be made ahead of time and reheated in the oven or air fryer before serving.
- To make this recipe gluten-free, use a gluten-free all-purpose flour or ground flaxseed instead of the whole wheat flour.
- Serve the falafel with a side of roasted vegetables or a fresh salad for a complete diabetic-friendly meal.

These simple 4-ingredient baked falafel are a delicious and diabetic-friendly alternative to the traditional fried version. They provide a good source of plant-based protein and fiber to keep you feeling full and satisfied.

67. Tomato and Basil Salad

Ingredients:

- 2 cups cherry or grape tomatoes, halved
- 1/2 cup fresh basil leaves, chopped
- 2 tbsp balsamic vinegar
- 1 tsp olive oil

Instructions:

1. In a medium bowl, combine the halved cherry or grape tomatoes and chopped fresh basil leaves.

2. Drizzle the balsamic vinegar and olive oil over the tomato and basil mixture.

3. Gently toss the salad to evenly coat the ingredients with the vinaigrette.

4. Serve the tomato and basil salad immediately, or refrigerate it for 30 minutes to allow the flavors to meld.

Tips:
- For extra flavor, you can add a pinch of salt and black pepper to the salad.

- Swap the cherry or grape tomatoes for diced beefsteak or heirloom tomatoes if desired.

- This salad is also delicious with the addition of diced cucumber, red onion, or crumbled feta cheese.

- Serve the tomato and basil salad as a side dish or light main course. It pairs well with grilled chicken, fish, or roasted vegetables.

This simple 4-ingredient tomato and basil salad is a refreshing and diabetic-friendly option for a quick and easy side dish or light meal. The bright, tangy flavors of the balsamic vinaigrette complement the juicy tomatoes and fragrant basil perfectly.

Vegetarian and Vegan Dishes

PreparationTime: 10 minutes
Total Time: 10 minutes
Serves: 4

68. Zucchini Fritters

Ingredients:

- 2 medium zucchini, grated
- 1 egg, beaten
- 1/4 cup all-purpose flour
- 2 tablespoons grated Parmesan cheese
- 1 garlic clove, minced
- 1/4 teaspoon salt
- 1/4 teaspoon black pepper
- 2 tablespoons olive oil

Vegetarian and Vegan Dishes

PreparationTime: 10 minutes
Cook Time: 15 minutes
Total Time: 25 minutes
Serves: 4

Instructions:

1. Grate the zucchini using a box grater or food processor. Place the grated zucchini in a clean kitchen towel and squeeze out as much moisture as possible.

2. In a medium bowl, combine the grated zucchini, beaten egg, flour, Parmesan, garlic, salt, and pepper. Mix well until fully incorporated.

3. Heat the olive oil in a large skillet over medium heat.

4. Scoop heaping tablespoons of the zucchini mixture and gently place them in the hot oil, flattening slightly with a spatula.

5. Cook the fritters for 2-3 minutes per side, until golden brown.

6. Transfer the cooked fritters to a paper towel-lined plate.

7. Serve the zucchini fritters warm, garnished with additional Parmesan cheese or fresh herbs if desired.

Enjoy your homemade zucchini fritters!

69. Butternut Squash Soup

Ingredients:

- 1 medium butternut squash, peeled,
 seeded and cubed (about 4 cups)
- 4 cups low-sodium chicken or vegetable broth
- 1 teaspoon ground cinnamon
- 1/4 teaspoon ground nutmeg

PreparationTime: 10 minutes
Cook Time: 30 minutes
Total Time: 40 minutes
Serves: 4

Instructions:

1. In a large pot or Dutch oven, combine the cubed butternut squash and broth. Bring to a boil over high heat.

2. Once boiling, reduce heat to medium-low, cover and simmer for 25-30 minutes, until the squash is very soft.

3. Remove the pot from heat and use an immersion blender to puree the soup until smooth. Alternatively, you can carefully transfer the soup to a blender in batches and blend until smooth.

4. Stir in the cinnamon and nutmeg. Taste and adjust seasoning as needed.

5. Serve the butternut squash soup warm. Top with a sprinkle of cinnamon or a drizzle of olive oil if desired.

This simple 4-ingredient soup is naturally low in carbs and high in fiber, making it a great option for those managing diabetes. The cinnamon and nutmeg add warmth and depth of flavor without any added sugars.

Enjoy this comforting and healthy butternut squash soup!

70. Cucumber and Avocado Salad

Ingredients:

- 2 medium cucumbers, sliced
- 1 ripe avocado, diced
- 2 tablespoons olive oil
- 1 tablespoon lemon juice

Instructions:

1. In a large bowl, combine the sliced cucumbers and diced avocado.

2. Drizzle the olive oil and lemon juice over the top.

3. Gently toss the salad to coat the cucumber and avocado evenly with the dressing.

4. Season with a pinch of salt and pepper, if desired.

5. Serve the cucumber and avocado salad immediately, or refrigerate until ready to serve.

This simple 4-ingredient salad is a great option for those managing diabetes. The healthy fats from the avocado and the low-carb cucumbers make it a nutritious and filling side dish or light meal.

The olive oil and lemon juice dressing provides flavor without any added sugars. This salad is refreshing, creamy, and perfect for hot summer days.

Enjoy this easy and diabetes-friendly cucumber and avocado salad!

Vegetarian and Vegan Dishes

PreparationTime: 10 minutes
Total Time: 10 minutes
Serves: 4

71. Chicken and Avocado Salad

Ingredients:

- 2 cups cooked, shredded chicken breast
- 1 ripe avocado, diced
- 2 tablespoons olive oil
- 1 tablespoon lemon juice

Instructions:

1. In a medium bowl, combine the shredded chicken and diced avocado.

2. Drizzle the olive oil and lemon juice over the top.

3. Gently toss the salad to coat the chicken and avocado evenly with the dressing.

4. Season with a pinch of salt and pepper, if desired.

5. Serve the chicken and avocado salad immediately, or refrigerate until ready to serve.

This simple 4-ingredient salad is a great option for those managing diabetes. The healthy fats from the avocado and the protein-rich chicken make it a nutritious and filling meal.

The olive oil and lemon juice dressing provides flavor without any added sugars. This salad is creamy, flavorful, and can be enjoyed on its own or served on a bed of greens.

Enjoy this easy and diabetes-friendly chicken and avocado salad!

More Dishes (Mixed Categories)

PreparationTime: 10 minutes
Total Time: 10 minutes
Serves: 4

72. Greek Salad

Ingredients:

- 1 cucumber, diced
- 1 pint cherry tomatoes, halved
- 1/2 cup crumbled feta cheese
- 2 tablespoons olive oil
- 1 tablespoon red wine vinegar

PreparationTime: 10 minutes
Total Time: 10 minutes
Serves: 4

Instructions:

1. In a large bowl, combine the diced cucumber and halved cherry tomatoes.

2. Sprinkle the crumbled feta cheese over the top.

3. In a small bowl, whisk together the olive oil and red wine vinegar to make the dressing.

4. Drizzle the dressing over the salad and gently toss to coat.

5. Serve the Greek salad immediately, or refrigerate until ready to serve.

This simple 4-ingredient Greek salad is a great option for those managing diabetes. The vegetables provide fiber and nutrients, while the feta cheese adds a creamy, tangy flavor.

The olive oil and red wine vinegar dressing is low in carbs and provides healthy fats without any added sugars. This salad is refreshing, flavorful, and can be enjoyed as a side dish or a light main course.

Enjoy this easy and diabetes-friendly Greek salad!

73. Almond Crusted Tilapia

Ingredients:

- 4 tilapia fillets (about 1 lb total)
- 1/2 cup sliced almonds
- 2 tablespoons grated Parmesan cheese
- 1 teaspoon dried parsley
- 1/4 teaspoon garlic powder
- 1/4 teaspoon salt
- 1/8 teaspoon black pepper
- 1 tablespoon olive oil

PreparationTime: 10 minutes
Cook Time: 15 minutes
Total Time: 25 minutes
Serves: 4

Instructions:

1. Preheat your oven to 400°F (200°C). Line a baking sheet with parchment paper.

2. In a shallow bowl, combine the sliced almonds, Parmesan cheese, dried parsley, garlic powder, salt, and black pepper. Mix well.

3. Pat the tilapia fillets dry with paper towels. Brush the top of each fillet lightly with olive oil.

4. Dip the oiled side of the tilapia into the almond mixture, pressing gently to help the coating adhere.

5. Place the almond-crusted tilapia fillets on the prepared baking sheet.

6. Bake for 12-15 minutes, or until the fish is cooked through and the crust is golden brown.

7. Serve the almond crusted tilapia immediately, garnished with additional parsley if desired.

This almond-crusted tilapia is a delicious and easy-to-make baked fish dish. The crunchy almond topping adds a wonderful texture and flavor to the tender, flaky tilapia. It's a healthy and satisfying meal that's perfect for weeknight dinners.

Enjoy your almond crusted tilapia!

74. Cauliflower Pizza Crust

Ingredients:

- 1 medium head of cauliflower,
cut into florets (about 4 cups riced)
- 1 egg, beaten
- 1/2 cup shredded mozzarella cheese
- 2 tablespoons grated Parmesan cheese
- 1/2 teaspoon dried oregano
- 1/4 teaspoon garlic powder
- 1/4 teaspoon salt

More Dishes (Mixed Categories)

PreparationTime: 15 minutes
Cook Time: 30 minutes
Total Time: 45 minutes
Serves: 4 (1 pizza crust)

Instructions:

1. Preheat your oven to 400°F (200°C). Line a baking sheet with parchment paper.

2. Place the cauliflower florets in a food processor and pulse until it resembles the texture of rice or couscous. You should have about 4 cups of riced cauliflower.

3. Transfer the riced cauliflower to a microwave-safe bowl and microwave for 5-7 minutes, until tender. Allow to cool slightly.

4. Once cooled, place the riced cauliflower in a clean kitchen towel or cheesecloth and squeeze out as much moisture as possible. This is an important step to ensure a crispy crust.

5. In a medium bowl, combine the squeezed cauliflower, beaten egg, mozzarella, Parmesan, oregano, garlic powder, and salt. Mix well until fully incorporated.

6. Transfer the cauliflower mixture to the prepared baking sheet and press it into a thin, even circle, about 1/4-inch thick.

7. Bake the cauliflower crust for 25-30 minutes, until golden brown and crispy.

8. Remove the crust from the oven and top with your desired pizza toppings. Return the pizza to the oven and bake for an additional 10-15 minutes, until the toppings are heated through and the cheese is melted.

9. Slice and serve the cauliflower pizza crust immediately.

Enjoy your homemade, low-carb cauliflower pizza crust!

75. Spinach and Ricotta Stuffed Shells

Ingredients:

- 12 jumbo pasta shells
- 1 (15 oz) container part-skim ricotta cheese
- 1 (10 oz) package frozen chopped spinach,
 thawed and squeezed dry
- 1/4 cup grated Parmesan cheese

More Dishes (Mixed Categories)

PreparationTime: 20 minutes
Cook Time: 25 minutes
Total Time: 45 minutes
Serves: 4 (3 stuffed shells per serving)

Instructions:

1. Preheat your oven to 375°F (190°C). Grease a 9x13 inch baking dish.

2. Cook the pasta shells according to package instructions until al dente. Drain and set aside.

3. In a medium bowl, mix together the ricotta cheese, thawed and drained spinach, and Parmesan cheese until well combined.

4. Stuff each cooked pasta shell with a heaping tablespoon of the ricotta-spinach mixture.

5. Arrange the stuffed shells in the prepared baking dish.

6. Bake for 20-25 minutes, until the shells are heated through and the cheese is melted.

7. Serve the spinach and ricotta stuffed shells warm.

This simple 4-ingredient recipe is a great option for those managing diabetes. The ricotta cheese and spinach provide protein and fiber, while the Parmesan cheese adds flavor without any added sugars.

The stuffed shells make a satisfying and nutritious meal or side dish. Pair them with a fresh salad for a complete diabetic-friendly dinner.

Enjoy these easy and diabetes-friendly spinach and ricotta stuffed shells!

76. Avocado Deviled Eggs

Ingredients:

- 6 hard-boiled eggs, peeled and halved
- 1 ripe avocado, mashed
- 1 tablespoon lemon juice
- 1/4 teaspoon salt

Instructions:

1. Carefully scoop out the yolks from the hard-boiled egg halves and place them in a medium bowl.

2. Add the mashed avocado, lemon juice, and salt to the bowl with the egg yolks. Mash and mix everything together until well combined and creamy.

3. Spoon or pipe the avocado-yolk mixture back into the egg white halves.

4. Arrange the filled egg halves on a serving platter.

5. Refrigerate the avocado deviled eggs until ready to serve.

This simple 4-ingredient recipe is a great option for those managing diabetes. The healthy fats from the avocado provide creaminess and nutrition, while the lemon juice and salt add flavor without any added sugars.

Avocado deviled eggs make a delicious and satisfying snack or appetizer. They are low in carbs and high in protein, making them a great choice for those following a diabetic-friendly diet.

Enjoy these easy and diabetes-friendly avocado deviled eggs!

More Dishes (Mixed Categories)

PreparationTime: 15 minutes
Total Time: 15 minutes
Serves: 12 (2 halves per serving)

77. Turkey and Spinach Stuffed Mushrooms

Ingredients:

- 24 medium cremini or button mushrooms, stems removed and finely chopped
- 1 lb ground turkey
- 2 cups fresh spinach, chopped
- 1/4 cup grated Parmesan cheese
- 1/4 teaspoon garlic powder
- 1/4 teaspoon salt
- 1/8 teaspoon black pepper

More Dishes (Mixed Categories)

PreparationTime: 15 minutes
Cook Time: 20 minutes
Total Time: 35 minutes
Serves: 12 (2 stuffed mushrooms per serving)

Instructions:

1. Preheat your oven to 375°F (190°C). Line a baking sheet with parchment paper.

2. Remove the stems from the mushrooms and finely chop them. Set the mushroom caps aside.

3. In a skillet over medium heat, cook the ground turkey, breaking it up as it cooks, until no longer pink, about 5-7 minutes. Drain any excess fat.

4. Add the chopped mushroom stems, spinach, Parmesan, garlic powder, salt, and pepper to the cooked turkey. Stir to combine and cook for an additional 2-3 minutes, until the spinach is wilted.

5. Spoon the turkey and spinach mixture into the mushroom caps, packing it in gently.

6. Arrange the stuffed mushrooms on the prepared baking sheet.

7. Bake for 15-20 minutes, until the mushrooms are tender and the filling is hot.

8. Serve the turkey and spinach stuffed mushrooms warm.

These stuffed mushrooms make a delicious and healthy appetizer or snack. The combination of ground turkey, spinach, and Parmesan creates a flavorful and satisfying filling.

Enjoy these turkey and spinach stuffed mushrooms!

78. Zoodles with Tomato Sauce

Ingredients:

- 4 medium zucchini, spiralized into zoodles
- 1 (14 oz) can diced tomatoes
- 2 cloves garlic, minced
- 2 tablespoons olive oil

Instructions:

1. In a large skillet, heat the olive oil over medium heat. Add the minced garlic and cook for 1 minute, until fragrant.

2. Add the can of diced tomatoes (with their juices) to the skillet. Bring the sauce to a simmer and cook for 5-7 minutes, stirring occasionally, until slightly thickened.

3. Add the spiralized zucchini noodles (zoodles) to the skillet and toss to coat with the tomato sauce. Cook for an additional 5-7 minutes, until the zoodles are tender but still have a bit of bite.

4. Season the zoodles and tomato sauce with a pinch of salt and pepper, to taste.

5. Serve the zoodles with tomato sauce immediately, garnished with fresh basil or Parmesan cheese if desired.

This 4-ingredient recipe is a great option for those managing diabetes. Zucchini noodles are low in carbs and high in fiber, making them a healthier alternative to traditional pasta. The simple tomato sauce provides flavor without any added sugars.

This dish is quick, easy, and packed with nutrients. Enjoy this delicious and diabetes-friendly zoodles with tomato sauce!

More Dishes (Mixed Categories)

PreparationTime: 10 minutes
Cook Time: 15 minutes
Total Time: 25 minutes
Serves: 4

79. Baked Eggs in Avocado

Ingredients:

- 1 ripe avocado, halved and pitted
- 4 eggs
- 2 tablespoons grated Parmesan cheese
- Salt and pepper to taste
- Chopped fresh parsley for garnish (optional)

PreparationTime: 10 minutes
Cook Time: 15 minutes
Total Time: 25 minutes
Serves: 2

Instructions:

1. Preheat your oven to 425°F (220°C). Line a baking sheet with parchment paper.

2. Carefully scoop out a little more of the avocado flesh from the center of each avocado half, creating a larger well to hold the egg.

3. Crack one egg into each avocado half, being careful not to break the yolk.

4. Sprinkle the grated Parmesan cheese over the top of the eggs.

5. Season with salt and pepper to taste.

6. Bake the stuffed avocado halves for 12-15 minutes, or until the egg whites are set and the yolks are cooked to your desired doneness.

7. Carefully remove the baked avocado halves from the oven and transfer them to a serving plate.

8. Garnish with chopped fresh parsley, if desired.

9. Serve the baked eggs in avocado immediately, while hot.

This simple and nutritious dish combines the healthy fats of avocado with the protein-rich eggs. It's a great option for a low-carb, keto-friendly breakfast or brunch.

Enjoy your baked eggs in avocado!

80. Caprese Salad

Ingredients:

- 8 oz fresh mozzarella cheese, sliced
- 1 pint cherry tomatoes, halved
- 1/4 cup fresh basil leaves, torn or chopped
- 2 tablespoons balsamic glaze

Instructions:

1. Arrange the sliced mozzarella cheese and halved cherry tomatoes on a serving platter or plate.

2. Sprinkle the torn or chopped fresh basil leaves over the top.

3. Drizzle the balsamic glaze over the salad.

4. Season with a pinch of salt and pepper, if desired.

5. Serve the Caprese salad immediately.

This simple 4-ingredient Caprese salad is a great option for those managing diabetes. The fresh mozzarella cheese and tomatoes provide a good source of protein and nutrients, while the basil and balsamic glaze add flavor without any added sugars.

The Caprese salad is a refreshing and light dish that can be enjoyed as a side or a main course. It's perfect for hot summer days or as a healthy appetizer.

Enjoy this easy and diabetes-friendly Caprese salad!

More Dishes (Mixed Categories)

PreparationTime: 10 minutes
Total Time: 10 minutes
Serves: 4

81. Salmon and Asparagus Foil Packets

Ingredients:

- 4 (4 oz) salmon fillets
- 1 lb asparagus, trimmed
- 2 tablespoons olive oil
- 1/4 teaspoon salt

Instructions:

1. Preheat your oven to 400°F (200°C).

2. Tear off four 12-inch squares of heavy-duty aluminum foil.

3. Place one salmon fillet in the center of each foil square. Top each salmon fillet with a quarter of the asparagus spears.

4. Drizzle the olive oil over the salmon and asparagus, and sprinkle with the salt.

5. Fold the foil over the salmon and asparagus, and crimp the edges to seal the packets.

6. Place the foil packets on a baking sheet and bake for 18-20 minutes, until the salmon is cooked through and the asparagus is tender.

7. Carefully open the foil packets and serve the salmon and asparagus immediately.

This simple 4-ingredient recipe is a great option for those managing diabetes. The salmon provides heart-healthy omega-3 fatty acids, while the asparagus is low in carbs and high in fiber.

The foil packet cooking method helps to retain the natural flavors and nutrients of the ingredients. This dish is easy to prepare, clean up is a breeze, and it's a complete meal all in one.

Enjoy this delicious and diabetes-friendly salmon and asparagus foil packet!

More Dishes (Mixed Categories)

PreparationTime: 10 minutes
Cook Time: 20 minutes
Total Time: 30 minutes
Serves: 4

82. Baked Chicken Thighs with Herbs

Ingredients:

- 8 bone-in, skin-on chicken thighs
- 2 tablespoons olive oil
- 1 tablespoon dried Italian seasoning
- 1/2 teaspoon salt

PreparationTime: 5 minutes
Cook Time: 40 minutes
Total Time: 45 minutes
Serves: 4

Instructions:

1. Preheat your oven to 400°F (200°C). Line a baking sheet with parchment paper.

2. Pat the chicken thighs dry with paper towels and place them on the prepared baking sheet.

3. Drizzle the olive oil over the chicken thighs and use your hands to evenly coat them.

4. Sprinkle the dried Italian seasoning and salt over the chicken, rubbing it in to ensure even coverage.

5. Bake the chicken thighs for 35-40 minutes, or until the internal temperature reaches 165°F (75°C) and the skin is crispy.

6. Remove the baked chicken thighs from the oven and let them rest for 5 minutes before serving.

This simple 4-ingredient recipe is a great option for those managing diabetes. Chicken thighs are a flavorful and affordable cut of meat that is low in carbs and high in protein.

The olive oil, Italian seasoning, and salt provide plenty of flavor without any added sugars. This dish is easy to prepare and makes a satisfying, diabetes-friendly meal.

Serve the baked chicken thighs with a side of roasted vegetables or a fresh salad for a complete and nutritious dinner.

Enjoy this delicious and diabetes-friendly baked chicken thighs with herbs!

83. Seared Scallops with Spinach

Ingredients:

- 1 lb sea scallops, patted dry
- 2 tablespoons olive oil
- 4 cups fresh spinach leaves
- 1 tablespoon lemon juice

PreparationTime: 10 minutes
Cook Time: 10 minutes
Total Time: 20 minutes
Serves: 4

Instructions:

1. Heat a large skillet over high heat. Add the olive oil.

2. Season the scallops with a pinch of salt and pepper. Working in batches if needed, sear the scallops for 2-3 minutes per side, until golden brown. Transfer the seared scallops to a plate.

3. Reduce the heat to medium and add the fresh spinach leaves to the same skillet. Cook the spinach, stirring frequently, until wilted, about 2-3 minutes.

4. Remove the skillet from heat and stir in the lemon juice. Season the spinach with a pinch of salt and pepper.

5. Divide the wilted spinach among serving plates. Top with the seared scallops.

6. Serve the seared scallops with spinach immediately.

This simple 4-ingredient recipe is a great option for those managing diabetes. Scallops are a lean protein that is low in carbs, while the spinach provides fiber and nutrients.

The quick searing method helps to keep the scallops tender and juicy, while the lemon juice adds a bright, tangy flavor without any added sugars.

Enjoy this delicious and diabetes-friendly seared scallops with spinach dish!

84. Garlic Butter Shrimp

Ingredients:

- 1 lb large shrimp, peeled and deveined
- 2 tablespoons unsalted butter
- 2 cloves garlic, minced
- 1 tablespoon lemon juice

More Dishes (Mixed Categories)

PreparationTime: 5 minutes
Cook Time: 10 minutes
Total Time: 15 minutes
Serves: 4

Instructions:

1. In a large skillet, melt the butter over medium heat.

2. Add the minced garlic to the melted butter and cook for 1 minute, until fragrant.

3. Add the shrimp to the skillet and cook for 3-5 minutes, stirring occasionally, until the shrimp are pink and cooked through.

4. Remove the skillet from heat and stir in the lemon juice. Season with a pinch of salt and pepper, to taste.

5. Serve the garlic butter shrimp immediately, garnished with chopped parsley if desired.

This simple 4-ingredient recipe is a great option for those managing diabetes. Shrimp is a lean protein that is low in carbs, while the garlic, butter, and lemon provide flavor without any added sugars.

The quick cooking time helps to preserve the natural sweetness and texture of the shrimp. This dish is easy to prepare and makes a delicious, diabetes-friendly meal or appetizer.

Serve the garlic butter shrimp over a bed of zucchini noodles or with a side salad for a complete and satisfying dinner.

Enjoy this flavorful and diabetes-friendly garlic butter shrimp!

85. Chicken and Broccoli Stir-Fry

Ingredients:

- 1 lb boneless, skinless chicken breasts,
cut into 1-inch pieces
- 1 head of broccoli,
cut into florets (about 4 cups)
- 2 tablespoons low-sodium soy sauce
- 1 tablespoon sesame oil

PreparationTime: 10 minutes
Cook Time: 15 minutes
Total Time: 25 minutes
Serves: 4

Instructions:

1. Heat a large skillet or wok over high heat. Add the sesame oil and swirl to coat the bottom of the pan.

2. Add the chicken pieces to the hot pan and stir-fry for 5-7 minutes, until the chicken is cooked through and no longer pink.

3. Add the broccoli florets to the pan and continue to stir-fry for an additional 5-7 minutes, until the broccoli is tender-crisp.

4. Drizzle the low-sodium soy sauce over the chicken and broccoli, and toss to coat everything evenly.

5. Serve the chicken and broccoli stir-fry immediately, while hot.

This simple 4-ingredient recipe is a great option for those managing diabetes. Chicken is a lean protein, while broccoli is a low-carb vegetable that is high in fiber and nutrients.

The soy sauce and sesame oil provide flavor without any added sugars. This dish is quick and easy to prepare, making it a perfect weeknight meal.

Serve the chicken and broccoli stir-fry over a bed of cauliflower rice or zucchini noodles for a complete, diabetes-friendly meal.

Enjoy this delicious and healthy chicken and broccoli stir-fry!

86. Lemon Garlic Tilapia

Ingredients:

- 4 (4 oz) tilapia fillets
- 2 tablespoons olive oil
- 2 tablespoons lemon juice
- 2 cloves garlic, minced

PreparationTime: 5 minutes
Cook Time: 15 minutes
Total Time: 20 minutes
Serves: 4

Instructions:

1. Preheat your oven to 400°F (200°C). Line a baking sheet with parchment paper.

2. Place the tilapia fillets on the prepared baking sheet.

3. In a small bowl, whisk together the olive oil, lemon juice, and minced garlic.

4. Drizzle the lemon-garlic mixture evenly over the top of the tilapia fillets.

5. Bake for 12-15 minutes, or until the fish is cooked through and flakes easily with a fork.

6. Serve the lemon garlic tilapia immediately, garnished with fresh parsley or lemon wedges if desired.

This simple 4-ingredient recipe is a great option for those managing diabetes. Tilapia is a lean, mild-flavored fish that is low in carbs and high in protein. The lemon and garlic provide flavor without any added sugars.

The baked preparation method is easy and healthy, making this a quick and satisfying weeknight meal. Serve the lemon garlic tilapia with a side of roasted vegetables or a fresh salad for a complete diabetic-friendly dinner.

Enjoy this delicious and diabetes-friendly lemon garlic tilapia!

87. Balsamic Chicken and Tomatoes

Ingredients:

- 1 lb boneless, skinless chicken breasts,
cut into 1-inch pieces
- 2 tbsp olive oil
- 1 pint cherry or grape tomatoes, halved
- 2 cloves garlic, minced
- 2 tbsp balsamic vinegar
- 1 tsp dried oregano
- 1/4 tsp salt
- 1/4 tsp black pepper
- 2 tbsp chopped fresh basil (optional)

PreparationTime: 10 minutes
Cook Time: 20 minutes
Total Time: 30 minutes
Serves: 4

Instructions:

1. In a large skillet, heat the olive oil over medium-high heat. Add the chicken and cook for 5-7 minutes, stirring occasionally, until the chicken is lightly browned.

2. Add the tomatoes, garlic, balsamic vinegar, oregano, salt, and pepper. Stir to combine.

3. Reduce heat to medium-low and simmer for 10-12 minutes, stirring occasionally, until the chicken is cooked through and the tomatoes have softened.

4. Remove from heat and stir in the fresh basil, if using.

5. Serve immediately, over cooked pasta, rice, or with a side salad.

This dish is a quick and easy way to get a healthy, flavorful meal on the table. The balsamic vinegar and tomatoes create a delicious sauce that complements the tender chicken.

88. Ground Turkey and Zucchini Skillet

Ingredients:

- 1 lb ground turkey
- 2 medium zucchini, sliced
- 1 tsp garlic powder
- 1/2 tsp salt

Instructions:

1. In a large skillet over medium-high heat, cook the ground turkey, breaking it up as it cooks, until no longer pink, about 5-7 minutes.

2. Add the sliced zucchini, garlic powder, and salt. Stir to combine.

3. Continue cooking, stirring occasionally, until the zucchini is tender, about 5-7 more minutes.

4. Serve immediately.

This simple skillet dish is low in carbs and high in protein, making it a great diabetes-friendly meal. The zucchini adds fiber and nutrients. You can adjust the seasoning to your taste preferences.

More Dishes (Mixed Categories)

PreparationTime: 5 minutes
Cook Time: 12 minutes
Total Time: 17 minutes
Serves: 4

89. Shrimp and Avocado Salad

Ingredients:

- 1 lb cooked shrimp, peeled and deveined
- 1 ripe avocado, diced
- 2 tablespoons olive oil
- 1 tablespoon lemon juice

PreparationTime: 10 minutes
Total Time: 10 minutes
Serves: 4

Instructions:

1. In a large bowl, combine the cooked shrimp and diced avocado.

2. Drizzle the olive oil and lemon juice over the shrimp and avocado.

3. Gently toss the salad to coat the shrimp and avocado evenly with the dressing.

4. Season with a pinch of salt and pepper, if desired.

5. Serve the shrimp and avocado salad immediately, or refrigerate until ready to serve.

This simple 4-ingredient salad is a great option for those managing diabetes. Shrimp is a lean protein that is low in carbs, while the avocado provides healthy fats and creaminess.

The olive oil and lemon juice dressing adds flavor without any added sugars. This salad is refreshing, satisfying, and can be enjoyed as a light main course or a side dish.

Enjoy this easy and diabetes-friendly shrimp and avocado salad!

90. Cauliflower and Cheese Soup

Ingredients:

- 1 head of cauliflower,
cut into florets (about 4 cups)
- 4 cups low-sodium chicken or
 vegetable broth
- 1 cup shredded cheddar cheese
- 1/2 tsp salt

More Dishes (Mixed Categories)

PreparationTime: 10 minutes
Cook Time: 20 minutes
Total Time: 30 minutes
Serves: 4

Instructions:

1. In a large pot, bring the chicken or vegetable broth to a boil over high heat.

2. Add the cauliflower florets, reduce heat to medium-low, and simmer for 15-20 minutes, or until the cauliflower is very tender.

3. Using an immersion blender or regular blender, puree the soup until smooth.

4. Return the pureed soup to the pot and stir in the shredded cheddar cheese and salt. Heat, stirring occasionally, until the cheese is melted and the soup is heated through.

5. Serve hot.

This simple 4-ingredient soup is a great option for a diabetes-friendly meal. The cauliflower provides fiber, vitamins, and minerals, while the cheddar cheese adds protein and creaminess. The small amount of salt can be adjusted to your taste preferences.

You can top the soup with additional shredded cheese, chopped chives, or a sprinkle of paprika for extra flavor. Enjoy this comforting and nutritious soup!

91. Cucumber Tomato Feta Salad

Ingredients:

- 2 cups diced cucumber
- 1 cup cherry or grape tomatoes, halved
- 1/2 cup crumbled feta cheese
- 2 tbsp olive oil

PreparationTime: 10 minutes
Total Time: 10 minutes
Serves: 4

Instructions:

1. In a large bowl, combine the diced cucumber, halved tomatoes, and crumbled feta cheese.

2. Drizzle the olive oil over the top and gently toss to coat.

3. Serve immediately or refrigerate until ready to serve.

This simple 4-ingredient salad is perfect for a light, refreshing, and diabetes-friendly side dish or snack. The cucumber and tomatoes provide hydration, fiber, and vitamins, while the feta cheese adds a creamy, tangy flavor. The olive oil helps the body absorb the fat-soluble vitamins in the vegetables.

This salad is easy to make and can be enjoyed on its own or paired with grilled chicken, fish, or a lean protein for a complete meal. Adjust the amounts of each ingredient to suit your taste preferences.

92. Almond Butter and Banana Smoothie

Ingredients:

- 1 ripe banana, frozen
- 2 tbsp almond butter
- 1 cup unsweetened almond milk
- 1 tsp honey (optional)

Instructions:

More Dishes (Mixed Categories)

PreparationTime: 5 minutes
Total Time: 5 minutes
Serves: 1

1. In a blender, combine the frozen banana, almond butter, almond milk, and honey (if using).

2. Blend on high speed until smooth and creamy, about 1 minute.

3. Pour into a glass and enjoy immediately.

This simple 4-ingredient smoothie is a great option for a quick, nutritious breakfast or snack. The banana provides natural sweetness and fiber, while the almond butter adds healthy fats and protein to keep you feeling full and satisfied.

The almond milk keeps the smoothie light and creamy without adding too many calories or carbs. The honey is optional, but can be added if you prefer a slightly sweeter taste.

This smoothie is perfect for those following a diabetes-friendly diet, as it is low in carbs and high in nutrients. Feel free to adjust the amounts of each ingredient to suit your taste preferences.

Enjoy this delicious and healthy Almond Butter and Banana Smoothie!

93. Roasted Brussels Sprouts with Bacon

Ingredients:

- 1 lb Brussels sprouts, trimmed and halved
- 2 tbsp olive oil
- 4 slices bacon, cooked and crumbled
- 1/4 tsp salt

Instructions:

1. Preheat the oven to 400°F.

2. In a large bowl, toss the Brussels sprouts with the olive oil and salt until well coated.

3. Spread the Brussels sprouts in a single layer on a baking sheet.

4. Roast for 15-20 minutes, stirring halfway, until the Brussels sprouts are tender and lightly browned.

5. Remove from the oven and sprinkle the crumbled bacon over the top.

6. Serve immediately.

This simple 4-ingredient recipe is perfect for a diabetes-friendly side dish. The Brussels sprouts provide fiber, vitamins, and minerals, while the bacon adds a savory, smoky flavor. The small amount of olive oil helps the sprouts roast to perfection. Enjoy!

More Dishes (Mixed Categories)

PreparationTime: 10 minutes
Cook Time: 20 minutes
Total Time: 30 minutes
Serves: 4

94. Chicken Lettuce Wraps

Ingredients:

- 1 lb ground chicken or turkey
- 2 tbsp hoisin sauce
- 1 tbsp rice vinegar
- 1 tsp sesame oil
- 8-10 large lettuce leaves (such as romaine or bibb)
- Chopped green onions, for garnish (optional)

PreparationTime: 10 minutes
Cook Time: 10 minutes
Total Time: 20 minutes
Serves: 4

Instructions:

1. In a large skillet or wok, cook the ground chicken or turkey over medium-high heat, breaking it up with a wooden spoon as it cooks, until no longer pink, about 5-7 minutes.

2. Drain any excess fat from the pan.

3. Stir in the hoisin sauce, rice vinegar, and sesame oil. Cook for an additional 2-3 minutes, stirring frequently, until the chicken is coated in the sauce.

4. Spoon the chicken mixture into the lettuce leaves.

5. Top with chopped green onions, if desired.

6. Serve immediately, allowing each person to assemble their own lettuce wraps.

These Chicken Lettuce Wraps are a delicious and healthy option for a quick meal or appetizer. The ground chicken or turkey provides lean protein, while the lettuce leaves act as a low-carb, high-fiber wrap. The hoisin sauce, rice vinegar, and sesame oil add a flavorful Asian-inspired twist.

You can customize the filling by adding diced vegetables, such as carrots, bell peppers, or water chestnuts. Serve with a side of steamed broccoli or a fresh salad for a complete, well-balanced meal.

Enjoy these easy and delicious Chicken Lettuce Wraps!

95. Greek Yogurt Chicken Salad

Ingredients:

- 2 cups cooked, shredded chicken
- 1 cup plain Greek yogurt
- 1/4 cup diced cucumber
- 2 tbsp chopped fresh dill
- 1/4 tsp salt
- 1/4 tsp black pepper

Instructions:

1. In a medium bowl, combine the shredded chicken, Greek yogurt, diced cucumber, chopped dill, salt, and black pepper. Stir until well mixed.

2. Serve the chicken salad on a bed of lettuce, in a whole wheat pita, or with whole grain crackers.

This Greek Yogurt Chicken Salad is a healthy and delicious option for a quick lunch or snack. The Greek yogurt provides a creamy texture and a boost of protein, while the cucumber and dill add freshness and flavor.

This recipe is perfect for those following a diabetes-friendly diet, as it is low in carbs and high in protein and healthy fats. You can adjust the amount of each ingredient to suit your taste preferences.

For added crunch, you can also mix in some chopped celery, toasted almonds, or diced bell peppers. Enjoy this versatile and nutritious Greek Yogurt Chicken Salad!

More Dishes (Mixed Categories)

PreparationTime: 10 minutes
Total Time: 10 minutes
Serves: 4

96. Baked Tofu with Soy Sauce

Ingredients:

- 1 block (14 oz) extra-firm tofu, drained and cut into 1-inch cubes
- 2 tbsp low-sodium soy sauce
- 1 tbsp sesame oil
- 1 tsp honey
- 1/4 tsp garlic powder
- 1/4 tsp ground ginger
- 1 tbsp sesame seeds (optional)

PreparationTime: 10 minutes
Cook Time: 25 minutes
Total Time: 35 minutes
Serves: 4

Instructions:

1. Preheat the oven to 400°F. Line a baking sheet with parchment paper.

2. In a medium bowl, whisk together the soy sauce, sesame oil, honey, garlic powder, and ground ginger.

3. Add the tofu cubes to the bowl and gently toss to coat them evenly in the sauce.

4. Arrange the tofu cubes in a single layer on the prepared baking sheet.

5. Bake for 20-25 minutes, flipping the tofu halfway through, until the tofu is crispy and golden brown.

6. Remove from the oven and sprinkle with sesame seeds, if using.

7. Serve hot, over a bed of steamed rice or with a side of roasted vegetables.

This Baked Tofu with Soy Sauce is a simple, flavorful, and diabetes-friendly dish. The tofu provides a good source of plant-based protein, while the soy sauce, sesame oil, and spices add a delicious Asian-inspired taste. The baking process gives the tofu a crispy texture.

Feel free to adjust the seasoning to your taste preferences. This recipe can also be made with firm or extra-firm tofu. Enjoy this healthy and satisfying tofu dish!

97. Grilled Vegetable Skewers

Ingredients:

- 1 zucchini, cut into 1-inch pieces
- 1 yellow squash, cut into 1-inch pieces
- 1 red bell pepper, cut into 1-inch pieces
- 1 red onion, cut into 1-inch pieces
- 8 oz mushrooms, halved
- 2 tbsp olive oil
- 1 tsp dried Italian seasoning
- 1/4 tsp salt
- 1/4 tsp black pepper

Instructions:

1. Preheat grill to medium-high heat.

2. In a large bowl, combine the zucchini, yellow squash, bell pepper, onion, and mushrooms. Drizzle with the olive oil and sprinkle with the Italian seasoning, salt, and black pepper. Toss to coat the vegetables evenly.

3. Thread the vegetables onto metal or wooden skewers, leaving a small space between each piece.

4. Grill the vegetable skewers for 12-15 minutes, turning occasionally, until the vegetables are tender and lightly charred.

5. Serve the grilled vegetable skewers immediately, garnished with fresh herbs if desired.

These Grilled Vegetable Skewers are a delicious and healthy side dish or main course. The variety of vegetables provides a range of vitamins, minerals, and fiber, while the grilling process adds a smoky, caramelized flavor.

This recipe is perfect for a diabetes-friendly diet, as it is low in carbs and high in nutrients. You can customize the vegetables used based on your preferences or what's in season.

Serve the grilled vegetable skewers with grilled chicken, fish, or tofu for a complete and balanced meal. Enjoy this easy and flavorful summer dish!

More Dishes (Mixed Categories)

PreparationTime: 15 minutes
Cook Time: 15 minutes
Total Time: 30 minutes
Serves: 4

98. Eggplant and Tomato Bake

Ingredients:

- 1 medium eggplant, cut into 1-inch cubes
- 2 cups cherry or grape tomatoes, halved
- 1 onion, diced
- 2 cloves garlic, minced
- 2 tbsp olive oil
- 1 tsp dried oregano
- 1/2 tsp salt
- 1/4 tsp black pepper
- 1/2 cup shredded mozzarella cheese

Instructions:

1. Preheat the oven to 375°F. Grease a 9x13-inch baking dish.

2. In a large bowl, combine the cubed eggplant, halved tomatoes, diced onion, and minced garlic. Drizzle with the olive oil and sprinkle with the oregano, salt, and black pepper. Toss to coat the vegetables evenly.

3. Transfer the vegetable mixture to the prepared baking dish and spread it out in an even layer.

4. Bake for 30-35 minutes, stirring halfway, until the eggplant is tender and the tomatoes have released their juices.

5. Remove the dish from the oven and sprinkle the shredded mozzarella cheese over the top.

6. Return the dish to the oven and bake for an additional 5-7 minutes, or until the cheese is melted and bubbly. Serve hot, garnished with fresh basil or parsley, if desired.

This Eggplant and Tomato Bake is a delicious and healthy vegetarian dish. The eggplant and tomatoes provide fiber, vitamins, and antioxidants, while the mozzarella cheese adds a creamy, melty element. It's a great option for a diabetes-friendly side dish or main course.

You can customize the recipe by adding other vegetables, such as zucchini or bell peppers, or by using different types of cheese. Enjoy this flavorful and satisfying Eggplant and Tomato Bake!

More Dishes (Mixed Categories)

PreparationTime: 15 minutes
Cook Time: 40 minutes
Total Time: 55 minutes
Serves: 4

99. Spinach and Goat Cheese Stuffed Chicken

Ingredients:

- 4 boneless, skinless chicken breasts
- 4 oz goat cheese, softened
- 2 cups fresh spinach, chopped
- 2 cloves garlic, minced
- 1/4 tsp salt
- 1/4 tsp black pepper

More Dishes (Mixed Categories)

PreparationTime: 15 minutes
Cook Time: 30 minutes
Total Time: 45 minutes
Serves: 4

Instructions:

1. Preheat the oven to 375°F. Grease a baking dish or line a baking sheet with parchment paper.

2. In a medium bowl, mix together the goat cheese, chopped spinach, minced garlic, salt, and black pepper until well combined.

3. Using a sharp knife, cut a pocket into the side of each chicken breast, being careful not to cut all the way through.

4. Stuff each chicken breast with about 2-3 tablespoons of the spinach and goat cheese mixture, pressing it into the pocket.

5. Place the stuffed chicken breasts in the prepared baking dish or on the baking sheet.

6. Bake for 25-30 minutes, or until the chicken is cooked through and the internal temperature reaches 165°F.

7. Serve the Spinach and Goat Cheese Stuffed Chicken immediately.

This dish is a delicious and healthy option for a diabetes-friendly meal. The spinach provides fiber, vitamins, and minerals, while the goat cheese adds a creamy, tangy flavor. The chicken breast is a lean protein source.

You can serve the stuffed chicken with a side of roasted vegetables or a fresh salad for a complete and balanced meal. Enjoy this flavorful and satisfying Spinach and Goat Cheese Stuffed Chicken!

100. Lemon Dill Salmon

Ingredients:

- 4 (4 oz) salmon fillets
- 2 tbsp fresh dill, chopped
- 1 tbsp lemon juice
- 1/4 tsp salt

PreparationTime: 5 minutes
Cook Time: 15 minutes
Total Time: 20 minutes
Serves: 4

Instructions:

1. Preheat the oven to 400°F. Line a baking sheet with parchment paper.

2. Place the salmon fillets on the prepared baking sheet.

3. In a small bowl, mix together the chopped fresh dill, lemon juice, and salt.

4. Spoon the dill-lemon mixture evenly over the top of the salmon fillets, spreading it to cover the surface.

5. Bake for 12-15 minutes, or until the salmon is cooked through and flakes easily with a fork.

6. Serve the Lemon Dill Salmon immediately.

This simple 4-ingredient recipe is perfect for a diabetes-friendly meal. The salmon provides heart-healthy omega-3 fatty acids, while the fresh dill and lemon juice add a bright, flavorful topping.

The small amount of salt can be adjusted to your taste preferences. You can serve the Lemon Dill Salmon with a side of roasted vegetables or a fresh salad for a complete and balanced meal.

This dish is easy to prepare and makes for a delicious and nutritious dinner option. Enjoy this Lemon Dill Salmon!

101. Zucchini and Tomato Gratin

Ingredients:

- 2 medium zucchini, sliced into 1/4-inch rounds
- 2 cups cherry or grape tomatoes, halved
- 1/2 cup shredded mozzarella cheese
- 1/4 tsp salt

More Dishes (Mixed Categories)

PreparationTime: 10 minutes
Cook Time: 30 minutes
Total Time: 40 minutes
Serves: 4

Instructions:

1. Preheat the oven to 375°F. Grease a 9x13-inch baking dish.

2. Arrange the zucchini slices in a single layer in the prepared baking dish. Top with the halved tomatoes, spreading them out evenly.

3. Sprinkle the shredded mozzarella cheese over the top.

4. Season with the salt.

5. Bake for 25-30 minutes, or until the zucchini is tender and the cheese is melted and bubbly.

6. Serve hot.

This simple 4-ingredient Zucchini and Tomato Gratin is a great diabetes-friendly side dish or light main course. The zucchini and tomatoes provide fiber, vitamins, and antioxidants, while the mozzarella cheese adds a creamy, melty element.

You can customize the recipe by adding other herbs or spices, such as dried basil, garlic powder, or black pepper. For a heartier meal, you can also add cooked ground turkey or chicken.

This dish is easy to prepare and perfect for a weeknight dinner. Enjoy this delicious and nutritious Zucchini and Tomato Gratin!

102. Garlic Parmesan Cauliflower

Ingredients:

- 1 head of cauliflower,
cut into florets (about 4 cups)
- 2 tbsp olive oil
- 2 cloves garlic, minced
- 1/2 cup grated Parmesan cheese

Instructions:

1. Preheat the oven to 400°F. Line a baking sheet with parchment paper.

2. In a large bowl, toss the cauliflower florets with the olive oil and minced garlic until the cauliflower is evenly coated.

3. Spread the cauliflower in a single layer on the prepared baking sheet.

4. Sprinkle the grated Parmesan cheese evenly over the top of the cauliflower.

5. Bake for 18-22 minutes, or until the cauliflower is tender and the Parmesan is melted and lightly browned.

6. Serve hot.

This Garlic Parmesan Cauliflower is a simple and delicious side dish that is perfect for a diabetes-friendly diet. The cauliflower provides fiber, vitamins, and minerals, while the Parmesan cheese adds a savory, nutty flavor.

The garlic and olive oil help to enhance the overall taste and texture of the dish. This recipe is easy to prepare and can be enjoyed as a side or even as a snack.

You can adjust the amount of Parmesan cheese to suit your taste preferences. Additionally, you can add a sprinkle of dried herbs, such as oregano or basil, for extra flavor.

Enjoy this flavorful and healthy Garlic Parmesan Cauliflower!

More Dishes (Mixed Categories)

PreparationTime: 10 minutes
Cook Time: 20 minutes
Total Time: 30 minutes
Serves: 4

103. Chicken Zoodle Soup

Ingredients:

- 4 cups low-sodium chicken broth
- 2 cups shredded cooked chicken
- 2 medium zucchini, spiralized or julienned into noodles
- 1 cup sliced mushrooms
- 1/2 cup diced onion
- 2 cloves garlic, minced
- 1 tsp dried thyme
- 1/4 tsp salt
- 1/4 tsp black pepper
- 2 tbsp chopped fresh parsley (optional)

PreparationTime: 15 minutes
Cook Time: 30 minutes
Total Time: 45 minutes
Serves: 4

Instructions:

1. In a large pot, bring the chicken broth to a simmer over medium heat.

2. Add the shredded cooked chicken, zucchini noodles, sliced mushrooms, diced onion, and minced garlic.

3. Stir in the dried thyme, salt, and black pepper.

4. Simmer the soup for 20-25 minutes, or until the vegetables are tender.

5. Remove from heat and stir in the chopped fresh parsley, if using.

6. Serve the Chicken Zoodle Soup hot.

This Chicken Zoodle Soup is a delicious and diabetes-friendly option. The zucchini noodles provide a low-carb alternative to traditional pasta, while the chicken, mushrooms, and onions add protein and flavor.

The broth is low in sodium, making this a great choice for those watching their salt intake. You can customize the soup by adding other vegetables, such as spinach or bell peppers, or by using different herbs and spices.

Enjoy this comforting and nutritious Chicken Zoodle Soup!

104. Broccoli and Cheese Stuffed Chicken Breast

Ingredients:

- 4 boneless, skinless chicken breasts
- 1 cup chopped broccoli florets
- 1/2 cup shredded cheddar cheese
- 2 tbsp cream cheese, softened
- 1 clove garlic, minced
- 1/4 tsp salt
- 1/4 tsp black pepper

PreparationTime: 15 minutes
Cook Time: 30 minutes
Total Time: 45 minutes
Serves: 4

Instructions:

1. Preheat the oven to 375°F. Grease a baking dish or line a baking sheet with parchment paper.

2. In a medium bowl, mix together the chopped broccoli, shredded cheddar cheese, cream cheese, minced garlic, salt, and black pepper until well combined.

3. Using a sharp knife, cut a pocket into the side of each chicken breast, being careful not to cut all the way through.

4. Stuff each chicken breast with about 2-3 tablespoons of the broccoli and cheese mixture, pressing it into the pocket.

5. Place the stuffed chicken breasts in the prepared baking dish or on the baking sheet.

6. Bake for 25-30 minutes, or until the chicken is cooked through and the internal temperature reaches 165°F.

7. Serve the Broccoli and Cheese Stuffed Chicken Breast immediately.

This dish is a delicious and diabetes-friendly option. The broccoli provides fiber, vitamins, and minerals, while the cheese adds creaminess and protein. The chicken breast is a lean protein source.

You can serve the stuffed chicken with a side of roasted vegetables or a fresh salad for a complete and balanced meal. Enjoy this flavorful and satisfying Broccoli and Cheese Stuffed Chicken Breast!

105. Veggie and Hummus Wrap

Ingredients:

- 1 whole wheat tortilla or wrap
- 2 tbsp hummus
- 1/2 cup mixed vegetables
(such as sliced cucumber, shredded
 carrots, diced bell pepper)
- 1 tbsp crumbled feta cheese (optional)

Instructions:
1. Spread the hummus evenly over the tortilla or wrap.
2. Layer the mixed vegetables on top of the hummus.
3. Sprinkle the feta cheese over the vegetables, if using.
4. Fold the sides of the tortilla/wrap over the filling and roll up tightly.

Spinach and Feta Stuffed Peppers
Preparation Time: 15 minutes
Cook Time: 30 minutes
Total Time: 45 minutes
Serves: 4

Ingredients:
- 4 bell peppers, halved and seeded
- 1 cup chopped fresh spinach
- 1/2 cup crumbled feta cheese
- 2 tbsp diced onion
- 1 clove garlic, minced
- 1/4 tsp dried oregano
- 1/4 tsp salt
- 1/8 tsp black pepper

Instructions:
1. Preheat the oven to 375°F. Arrange the pepper halves in a baking dish.
2. In a bowl, mix together the spinach, feta cheese, onion, garlic, oregano, salt, and pepper.
3. Spoon the spinach-feta mixture evenly into the pepper halves.
4. Bake for 25-30 minutes, until the peppers are tender.
5. Serve the Spinach and Feta Stuffed Peppers warm.

Both of these recipes are diabetes-friendly, providing a balance of vegetables, protein, and healthy fats. Enjoy these delicious and nutritious options!

More Dishes (Mixed Categories)

PreparationTime: 10 minutes
Total Time: 10 minutes
Serves: 1

106. Almond Flour Pancakes

Ingredients:

- 1 cup almond flour
- 2 eggs
- 1/4 cup unsweetened almond milk
- 1 tsp baking powder
- 1/4 tsp salt
- 1 tsp vanilla extract (optional)

Instructions:

1. In a medium bowl, whisk together the almond flour, eggs, almond milk, baking powder, and salt until well combined. Stir in the vanilla extract if using.

2. Heat a non-stick skillet or griddle over medium heat. Grease the surface lightly with butter or non-stick cooking spray.

3. Scoop about 1/4 cup of the batter onto the hot surface, spreading it slightly to form a pancake shape.

4. Cook for 2-3 minutes per side, or until the pancakes are golden brown.

5. Repeat with the remaining batter, greasing the surface as needed.

6. Serve the almond flour pancakes warm, with your desired toppings such as fresh berries, a drizzle of sugar-free maple syrup, or a sprinkle of cinnamon.

These almond flour pancakes are a great diabetes-friendly breakfast option. Almond flour is low in carbs and high in healthy fats and protein, making it an excellent alternative to traditional wheat flour. The eggs also add protein to help keep blood sugar levels stable.

You can adjust the amount of almond milk to achieve your desired pancake consistency. Enjoy these delicious and nutritious Almond Flour Pancakes!

More Dishes (Mixed Categories)

PreparationTime: 10 minutes
Cook Time: 10 minutes
Total Time: 20 minutes
Serves: 4 (makes 8 pancakes)

107. Lemon Garlic Roasted Chicken

Ingredients:

- 1 (3-4 lb) whole chicken
- 2 tbsp olive oil
- 3 cloves garlic, minced
- 1 lemon, zested and juiced
- 1 tsp dried thyme
- 1 tsp salt
- 1/2 tsp black pepper

PreparationTime: 10 minutes
Cook Time: 60-75 minutes
Total Time: 70-85 minutes
Serves: 4

Instructions:

1. Preheat the oven to 400°F. Grease a large roasting pan or baking dish.

2. Pat the chicken dry with paper towels. Place the chicken in the prepared roasting pan.

3. In a small bowl, mix together the olive oil, minced garlic, lemon zest, lemon juice, dried thyme, salt, and black pepper.

4. Rub the lemon-garlic mixture all over the outside of the chicken, making sure to get it under the skin as well.

5. Roast the chicken for 60-75 minutes, or until the internal temperature reaches 165°F. Baste the chicken with the pan juices every 15 minutes.

6. Remove the chicken from the oven and let it rest for 10 minutes before carving and serving.

This Lemon Garlic Roasted Chicken is a delicious and diabetes-friendly main dish. The lemon and garlic provide bright, flavorful seasoning, while the olive oil and chicken provide healthy fats and protein.

Serve the roasted chicken with roasted vegetables or a fresh salad for a complete and balanced meal. The leftovers can also be used in other recipes, such as chicken salad or chicken soup.

Enjoy this easy and flavorful Lemon Garlic Roasted Chicken!

108. Spinach and Feta Stuffed Peppers

Ingredients:

- 4 bell peppers, halved and seeded
- 1 cup chopped fresh spinach
- 1/2 cup crumbled feta cheese
- 2 tbsp diced onion
- 1 clove garlic, minced
- 1/4 tsp dried oregano
- 1/4 tsp salt
- 1/8 tsp black pepper

More Dishes (Mixed Categories)

PreparationTime: 15 minutes
Cook Time: 30 minutes
Total Time: 45 minutes
Serves: 4

Instructions:

1. Preheat the oven to 375°F. Arrange the pepper halves in a baking dish.

2. In a medium bowl, mix together the chopped spinach, crumbled feta cheese, diced onion, minced garlic, dried oregano, salt, and black pepper.

3. Spoon the spinach-feta mixture evenly into the pepper halves.

4. Bake for 25-30 minutes, or until the peppers are tender.

5. Serve the Spinach and Feta Stuffed Peppers warm.

These Spinach and Feta Stuffed Peppers are a delicious and diabetes-friendly side dish or main course. The bell peppers provide fiber and vitamins, while the spinach and feta cheese add protein and healthy fats.

The combination of flavors is both satisfying and nutritious. You can adjust the amount of feta cheese or add other herbs and spices to suit your taste preferences.

Serve these Spinach and Feta Stuffed Peppers with a side salad or roasted vegetables for a complete and balanced meal. Enjoy this flavorful and healthy dish!

109. Turkey and Spinach Meatloaf

Ingredients:

- 1 lb ground turkey
- 1 cup chopped fresh spinach
- 1/2 cup diced onion
- 1 clove garlic, minced
- 1 egg
- 1/4 cup whole wheat breadcrumbs
- 2 tbsp tomato paste
- 1 tsp dried oregano
- 1/2 tsp salt
- 1/4 tsp black pepper

More Dishes (Mixed Categories)

PreparationTime: 15 minutes
Cook Time: 60 minutes
Total Time: 75 minutes
Serves: 6

Instructions:

1. Preheat the oven to 375°F. Grease a 9x5-inch loaf pan.

2. In a large bowl, combine the ground turkey, chopped spinach, diced onion, minced garlic, egg, breadcrumbs, tomato paste, oregano, salt, and black pepper. Mix until well incorporated.

3. Transfer the turkey mixture to the prepared loaf pan, pressing it down evenly.

4. Bake for 55-60 minutes, or until the internal temperature reaches 165°F.

5. Let the meatloaf rest for 10 minutes before slicing and serving.

This Turkey and Spinach Meatloaf is a delicious and diabetes-friendly main dish. The ground turkey provides lean protein, while the spinach adds fiber, vitamins, and minerals. The breadcrumbs help to bind the meatloaf together without adding too many carbs.

You can serve the meatloaf with roasted vegetables or a side salad for a complete and balanced meal. Leftovers can also be sliced and used in sandwiches or crumbled over a salad.

Enjoy this flavorful and nutritious Turkey and Spinach Meatloaf!

110. Avocado and Tomato Salad

Ingredients:

- 2 ripe avocados, diced
- 1 pint cherry or grape tomatoes, halved
- 1/4 cup diced red onion
- 2 tbsp fresh cilantro, chopped
- 1 tbsp olive oil
- 1 tbsp lime juice
- 1/4 tsp salt
- 1/8 tsp black pepper

Instructions:

1. In a large bowl, gently combine the diced avocados, halved tomatoes, diced red onion, and chopped cilantro.

2. Drizzle the olive oil and lime juice over the salad and season with salt and black pepper.

3. Toss the salad gently to coat the ingredients evenly.

4. Serve immediately or refrigerate until ready to serve.

This Avocado and Tomato Salad is a simple, refreshing, and diabetes-friendly dish. The avocado provides healthy fats, while the tomatoes and onion add fiber, vitamins, and antioxidants.

The olive oil and lime juice create a light, flavorful dressing that complements the fresh ingredients. You can adjust the amounts of each ingredient to suit your taste preferences.

This salad is a great option for a side dish or a light main course. Pair it with grilled chicken or fish for a complete and balanced meal. Enjoy this delicious and nutritious Avocado and Tomato Salad!

More Dishes (Mixed Categories)

PreparationTime: 10 minutes
Total Time: 10 minutes
Serves: 4